THE SAVVY TRAVELER'S GUIDE

to Homeopathy and Natural Medicine

Tips to Stay Healthy
Wherever You Go!

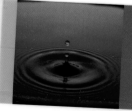

Abby Beale CCH RSHom(NA)

Certified Classical Homeopath

Office: 413-426-1024

Cell: 203-530-3367

HomeopathyHealings@gmail.com
www.HomeopathyHealings.com
~ *Offering Online Appointments* ~

ALSO BY THE AUTHORS

Homeopathic Self-Care

Whole Woman Homeopathy

Ritalin-Free Kids

Rage-Free Kids

The Homeopathic Treatment of
Depression, Anxiety, and Bipolar Disorder

A Drug-Free Approach to Asperger
Syndrome and Autism

The Patient's Guide to Homeopathic
Medicine

Mystics, Masters, Saints and Sages:
Stories of Enlightenment

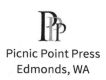

Picnic Point Press
Edmonds, WA

THE SAVVY TRAVELER'S GUIDE

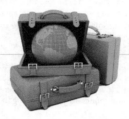

to Homeopathy and Natural Medicine

Tips to Stay Healthy Wherever You Go!

Judyth Reichenberg Ullman, N.D., M.S.W.
& Robert Ullman, N.D.

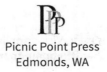

Picnic Point Press
Edmonds, WA

This book is intended for educational purposes only. It is not intended to diagnose, treat, or give medical advice for a specific condition, or in any way to replace the services of a qualified medical practitioner. The cases in this book are true stories from the authors' clinical practice, except where otherwise indicated. The names have been changed to protect confidentiality. Any names matching or resembling those of real people are coincidental and unintentional.

Book Design:	Ann Amberg
	www.annamberg.com
Published by:	Picnic Point Press
	123 4th Avenue N., Suite 2
	Edmonds, WA 98020
	(425) 774-5599

Library of Congress Cataloging-in-Publication Data

The savvy traveler's guide to homeopathy and natural medicine: tips to stay healthy wherever you go

236 pages

Includes bibliographical references.

ISBN 978-0-9640654-9-9

1. Homeopathy. 2. Travelers--Life skills guides.

RX76.S36 2014

615.5'32--dc23

2014002926

To Order: Visit us online at
www.healthyhomeopathy.com

*To all of those hardy, and at times foolhardy,
adventurers who have paved the way for our
travels to the middles and the ends of the earth.*

*To those helpful souls who have written travel
guidebooks and recommendations on Trip Advisor—
you have made our journeys far more informed,
insightful, comfortable and enjoyable.*

*To friends, old and new, named and unnamed,
familiar and foreign, who have opened to us their hearts
and homes. To patients, from many cultures, who have
trusted us to help them heal using natural medicine.*

*To all of our house sitters and pet sitters who have
freed us to travel, allowing us to rest easy that our
home and beloved pets were safe and loved.*

ACKNOWLEDGMENTS

A big "thank you" to Tom Blocher for his remarkable patience, persistence, good humor, inspiration, and innovative ideas. We feel so fortunate to call Ann Amberg our friend, neighbor, and book designer. Her creative and artful design talent, ease of communication, quick turnaround time, refreshing personality, and wealth of ideas have been invaluable. Our gratitude to Mary Aspinwall of Homeopathy World for designing the Homeopathy Specifics for the Traveler Kit, and for her encouragement in the initial phase of this project; and also to Joe Lillard of Washington Homeopathic Products for manufacturing our Homeopathic Self-Care Medicine Kit.

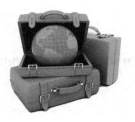

CONTENTS

Making the Most of Our User-Friendly Book

HOW THIS BOOK CAME TO BE

The very first, primitive version of this book was actually printed in 1984, shortly after the two of us met. **Judyth:** I was an avid backpacker and already a world traveler. I had just begun my naturopathic medical practice in Seattle and the two of us met at a homeopathic study group. **Bob:** I was new to Seattle, had been out of naturopathic school for a few years, had just met Judyth, and it was obvious that I had to become a hiker or the relationship would never last! Shortly after our meeting, we created a little blue booklet called *The Nature Cure Home Remedy Kit Guide,* reproduced at the local copy store. It came with a companion, blue rip-stop nylon kit with elastic loops to secure a dozen homeopathic medicines, six plastic bottles of herbs, and a webbed pocket for band-aids and other first aid paraphernalia.

Our original booklet contained 30 first aid conditions, along with basic instructions for homeopathic self-treatment, the use of *Calendula* and a few other tinctures, and acupressure points for each condition. We used it successfully for years, on our hiking and backpacking trips. Coincidentally, we recently reconnected with an old roommate of ours from that era, who, with his wife, found our booklet and kit, and later, *Homeopathic Self-Care,* to be indispensable in raising his children naturally.

The decades-long delay has given us time to accumulate considerably more personal and professional experience to share. We now live bi-continentally, dividing our year between the Pacific Northwest and the Lake District of Southern Chile. We remain avid, adventurous, off-the-beaten-path travelers. We are perpetually curious about, and fascinated by, the glorious rainbow of people and places on the planet. Awestruck by the diversity and magnificence of the natural world, we especially appreciate nature as one limitless homeopathic pharmacy of natural medicines. Now, thirty years

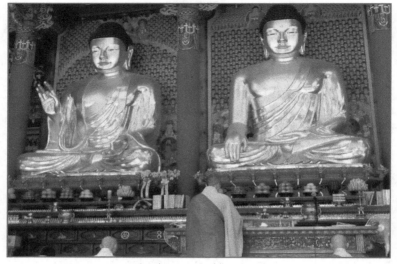

South Korean Buddhist Temple

later, after twenty-eight years of marriage, thirty-two years of naturopathic and homeopathic practice, travels to over forty countries, and eight books, this labor of love is coming to fruition.

WHY "SAVVY?"

We chose this word in our title because it captures what we most want to convey to you: practical knowledge, common sense, and wisdom. Savvy means sharp, perceptive, well informed, and intelligent. These qualities are essential for travel, because you will find yourself in situations that are new, unfamiliar, unpredictable, and challenging. Whether you are in Africa, with a ripped mosquito net and everyone around you speaking Swahili, or on a dark street in Quito being followed by a couple of menacing potential muggers, you need to have your wits about you. You may be a seasoned road warrior or are venturing out anew, and possibly alone. In either case, we invite you to benefit vicariously from our advice, some of it learned the hard way, to help ease your body, your mind, and your load (literally). Here's to happy, healthy, safe, and wonderful travels wherever you go!

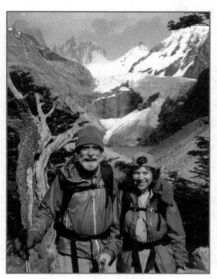

Torres del Paine National Park, Chile (recently voted The Eighth Wonder of the World)

HOW WE ORGANIZED THIS BOOK AND HOW TO USE IT

This book is filled with practical, user-friendly information that can make all the difference between enjoying your vacation or not. Even if you are already familiar with homeopathy, or you are a seasoned traveler, we hope you will learn valuable tidbits from our experience using homeopathy on the plane, on the trail or road, or even on a camel. Keep that kit handy!

No matter what your background and agenda, you will surely want to consult the **Travel Health Problems**, as they arise during your travels. If you suffer from a particular problem, you will want to read about it beforehand to prepare. If you do not yet have a travel kit, get one! Throughout our book, we include many references and links to resources, products, and services, which will hopefully ease your way.

Our goal is for you travel happily and healthily and to help your fellow travelers do the same. Although it is unrealistic to think you will stay healthy 100% of the time while traveling, this wealth of information can keep your down time to a minimum, if you go prepared and follow our recommendations.

The first chapters of the book provide practical information and tips on how to prepare for your trip, what to take and what to leave behind, how to prevent a variety of problems: such as getting sunburned, food-poisoned, or ripped off, and post-travel recommendations. Next we present homeopathy, with an emphasis on how to use it successfully for yourself and your travel companions, along with other down-to-earth natural tips.

How to Prepare for Your Trip

GET THAT BODY IN SHAPE

What a difference 10 to 30 extra pounds of fat can make when you're hiking the *Santiago de Compostela* pilgrimage trail, climbing Mt. Kilimanjaro, or climbing those endless steps to Mayan temples in Mexico and Guatemala!

- Use your upcoming trip as a perfect excuse to gear up your exercise program at home. Get help from a trainer, if necessary, to set up a challenging routine that will allow you to reach your weight loss goal. Add a Zumba, Body Pump, CrossFit, or other exercise class to firm your butt and tighten up those biceps.

- Walk as much as you can in airports before sitting for long hours.

- Pass on elevators and taxis and explore by foot. Not only will you do your heart and muscles a favor, but you will get much more of a taste of local flavor on the back streets than you ever will from a taxi.

- Pump and Tread on the Road: Many health clubs offer members a free pass to sister clubs throughout the U.S. and abroad.

- When booking your lodging, seek out jogging trails, bike paths with loaner cycles, gyms or exercise equipment.

- Pack a jump rope or other fitness gear that fits in a suitcase. www. nytimes.com/2012/04/28/travel/28iht-gear28.html?_r=0

AMP UP YOUR NATURAL IMMUNITY

The best way to stay well on your trip is to cultivate a wellness program way before your departure. The habits that you follow consecutively for 30 days are likely to become part on your ongoing routine. At least a month before leaving, begin:

- A healthy diet high in fresh, preferably organic, fruits and vegetables; whole grains (especially quinoa, brown rice, and oats); legumes (lentils and beans); fiber; wild salmon, halibut, and other omega-3 fish sources; organic dairy products and meat. Eliminate white sugar, artificial sweeteners and high-fructose corn syrup (HFCS). Change to honey, brown sugar, maple syrup, and stevia. Shop carefully to avoid ge-

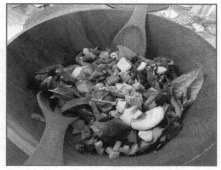

Organic greens from our Chilean huerta (garden)

netically modified (GMO) food items, particularly soy and corn. Minimize or eliminate caffeine and alcohol. Drink instead green tea, other herbal infusions, and plenty of good, old-fashioned water.

- Ingest lots more: fresh or frozen berries, almonds and walnuts, salads, tomatoes, broccoli and cabbage, apples, olive oil, citrus, and flaxseed.

- Try fruit and veggie smoothies for breakfast instead of bacon and eggs, salads rather than burgers for lunch, and a delicious and nutritious natural home-prepared meal, rather than a frozen, additives-laden TV dinner.

- Eat and savor SLOW rather than FAST foods.

- Maintain an ongoing healthy mega multi-vitamin and mineral supplement regimen.

- Have your serum Vitamin D levels tested. Make sure yours is at least in the low 40s, preferably the 50s or 60s. If not, take 2000-5000 IU until your levels come into range.

- Make sure you are getting enough dietary or supplemental calcium of high quality, such as citrate malate. This is even more important if you are thin, follow a demanding exercise program, have a family history of osteoporosis, take ongoing corticosteroids, or drink excessive amounts of alcohol or pop.

- Take a regular probiotic to maintain healthy gut flora or eat unsweetened yogurt.

TRAVEL WELL NATURAL TRAVEL HEALTH CONSULTATIONS

Pre-travel: Most travel consultations are orientated to conventional medicine, risk assessment and vaccinations, and are problem-oriented. Homeopathy and natural medicine stimulate your vital force and defense mechanism to keep you healthy. The goal of a natural health consult is to educate and empower you, given your individual concerns, predispositions, health concerns and challenges, and preferences. The best time to do this is six to eight weeks before traveling. There are various considerations to take into account:

- Special health issues such as pregnancy, breastfeeding, infancy or childhood, disability, immunity, age, surgery, or a recent or chronic significant health problem.

- A history of jet lag, motion sickness, altitude sickness, malaria, etc.

- Your dietary and natural medicine preferences.

- Your travel style—sedentary vs. diving, bungee jumping, rafting, climbing, hiking, cycling, kayaking, and extreme sports.

- How experienced a traveler you are and whether you are going alone.

- Exactly where you are going, for how long, and in which season.

- Preferred type of accommodations, diet on the road, comfort level, and tolerance for a lower level of hygiene than you are used to at home.

- Access to homeopathic medicines, herbs, nutritional supplements, and alternative and conventional health care during your travels.

- How well versed you are in taking care of your health naturally.

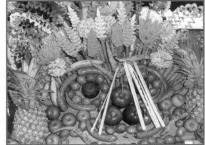

Balinese temple ceremonial fruit offering

During Your trip

Our book gives you much of what you need, but, if you become acutely ill with something that is beyond your self-help expertise, you can email drreichenberg@gmail.com or drbobullman@gmail.com or contact your natural health care provider at home, if available. For conventional travel health info in a pinch, you can access the CDC *Yel-*

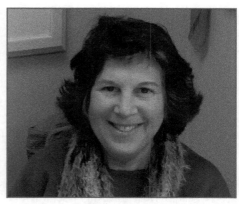

Dr. Reichenberg offers Travel Well consultations

low Book for International Travel 2014. www.cdc.gov But don't expect to read there about homeopathy and herbs. And we can't remind you often enough, pack your natural medicine kit!

Travel Vaccinations

It is a good idea to do your research long before you are due to travel. As with any medical intervention, weigh in on the risks and benefits. Research the latest online regarding recommendations and epidemics. Consult the CDC guidelines. nc.cdc.gov/travel/page/vaccinations

To ensure you get a balanced view, visit The National Vaccine Information Council, a watchdog organization that evaluates each vaccination individually to give you a good sense of the pros and cons. www.nvic.org/NVIC-site-search-result.aspx?q=travel%20immunizations

Consider:

- Risk of contracting the disease
- Severity of the disease
- Your track record of reactions to immunizations
- Where you are traveling
- What season of the year you are going

- How long you will be there
- Age
- Health and immune status
- Whether you will be staying in a rural or urban area
- Recent epidemics in the area
- Style of travel and accommodations
- Are you traveling with infants or small children?
- Are you pregnant?
- Are you a health care provider? Will you be working in hospitals or clinics while traveling? If so, where?

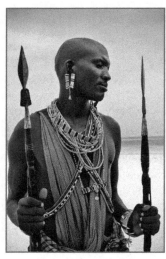

Maasai tribesman, Kenya

Only you can make the decision of whether or not to receive vaccinations, and which ones, for you and your family. Some vaccines may cause symptoms that are worse than the disease itself, and there are also increased risks involved in receiving vaccinations while visiting countries or continents (Africa) where hygiene standards may be questionable, and there is an increased risk of HIV and other infections. Some acute infectious diseases, generally of childhood, such as measles and chicken pox, may be better experienced than prevented in order to strengthen the immune system. A number of diseases for which vaccinations are recommended are readily treatable with homeopathy. If you do decide on vaccinations, ideally 4 to 6 weeks before travel, you can get them at your local public health department, a tropical medicine clinic, or from your doctor.

Some useful tips on the subject:

- "Routine" immunizations: We agree with tetanus vaccines every ten years, whether traveling or not, and dead polio vaccine. Diphtheria, also given once a decade, is still rampant in some lesser-developed countries and the former USSR.

- Smallpox is considered eradicated as of 1980, and immunizations are neither recommended nor available to the public.

- If you get a polio vaccine, a booster dose is recommended for adults once in their lifetime, and could be preventative in a travel destination where polio was present.

- Required vaccines: Yellow fever is prevalent in South America and Africa and is mosquito-transmitted. The mortality rate is 20% and there is no specific treatment in conventional medicine. Homeopathic treatment for yellow fever in the U.S. during 1800s reduced the mortality rate to 6%. The yellow fever vaccine is required to enter certain countries on those two continents. Adverse reactions have been reported in elderly travelers.

- Meningococcal (meningitis) vaccine may be necessary for visits to Saudi Arabia.

- Recommended vaccines: These are travel vaccines that may come up, depending on your destination: hepatitis A, hepatitis B, typhoid fever, meningococcal meningitis, cholera, flu, pneumococcal pneumonia, Japanese encephalitis, tick-borne encephalitis, rabies, and a TB skin test.

- Once you reach a border, you are at the mercy of the officials. Rumor has it that some Third World border officials look for opportunities to inject people with needles that may be far from sterile, and used many times previously. A certificate of exemption for the cholera vaccine may be required, even though it has not been legally required for many years in most countries.

We would be remiss if we did not mention homeopathic prophylaxis for travel (see Polio and Malaria). Homeopathy gained its claim to fame in the 1800s for outperforming any other kind of medicine in epidemics, such as cholera. We have avoided this controversial area in our practice, except for recommending homeopathic *Influenzinum* once a year, in the fall, which we have found to be effective for flu prevention.

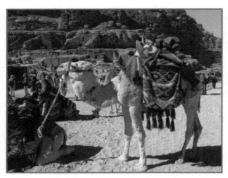

Camel in Petra, Jordan

HEDGING YOUR BETS AGAINST THE UNEXPECTED
Health Insurance

Regardless of age, accidents can happen. Many health insurance providers in the U.S. do cover emergencies while traveling, as do some Medicare supplemental plans. The insurers may require that the medical records be translated into English. Extreme-sport activities such as rock climbing, bungee jumping, paragliding, parasailing, and the like may be excluded. Certain plans, such as AirMed, cover emergency evacuation from a foreign hospital to one near your home. Do thorough research before traveling to avoid problems later.

Travel Insurance

The virtue of travel insurance is for unexpected changes in your travel plans. It may be more expensive than it is worth if you are flying on frequent-flyer miles and traveling independently, without making costly reservations in advance. It is most useful for prepaid, high-ticket items like cruises, tours, package trips, and pricey or inflexible air travel. These policies may also reimburse for trip interruption, delay, or cancellation, missed connections, baggage delay, or rental vehicle coverage, or even missed work. You can also opt for coverage of medical expenses, medical evacuation, and accidental death. The more protection you want, the more you pay.

CHECK OUT THE CLIMATE: METEOROLOGICAL AND POLITICAL

It takes a couple minutes to consult a 10-day weather forecast for your point(s) of destination, and that research can make the difference between being comfortable and sweltering, freezing, or being drenched. Global warming is changing climates throughout the world, and triggering natural disasters. In recent years, wherever we travel, we hear, "It didn't used to be this hot." Don't assume that the favorite place you visited 20 years ago will have the same climate now. Many of the glaciers in Glacier National Park in

Montana have lost their glacial ice, as have those in New Zealand. We hiked in Torres del Paine National Park in Chilean Patagonia eight years ago and again recently. Glacier Grey has receded two kilometers in the interim.

Check while planning your trip, and again just prior to leaving, for current travel advisories or danger zones. **Judyth:** I was one of the few American travelers who visited Egypt early in 2012, others being scared away by volatile demonstrations during the Arab Spring. I had a fabulous time, ran into no hostility, and benefited from great prices in the markets. I may have canceled my trip had I not been the guest of an Egyptian friend and her husband, who assured me that I would be perfectly safe. And so I was.

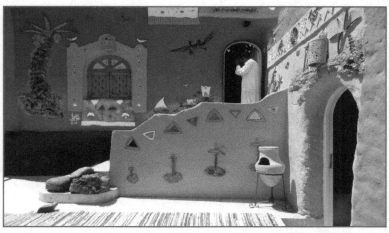

Sunny hotel in Aswan, Egypt

STIMULATE THOSE BRAIN CELLS—TRY A FOREIGN TONGUE

Besides opening yourself up to a whole new world of communication, depth of experience, and communication, learning a foreign language stimulates brain cells. Dr. Ellen Bialystok at York University found that dementia was delayed by four to five years in bilingual individuals. Speaking more than one language can widen your cultural world, enhance career opportunities, allow you to become more sensitive to cultural innuendos, and allow you to possibly even find a mate! Dive into an intensive language and cultural immersion program, a crash course online, CDs and DVDs, or even a foreign language television channel. Your travels will be richer and more rewarding.

MEDICAL TOURISM

A recent trend is to travel abroad to take care of medical needs that are either not available where you live, or are unaffordable. This type of journey clearly needs prior investigation and booking of appointments. Medical costs in the U.S. are exorbitant. Why not take care of your medical needs and enjoy a vacation at the same time? Medical tourists from developed countries travel to other countries with cheaper, yet equivalent care for a variety of procedures, both medical and cosmetic. These include treatment for cancer, dental issues, infertility and obesity. Also growing in popularity are international journeys for surgery, especially orthopedic procedures and even organ transplants. Prices in South America, India, Thailand, Eastern Europe and South Africa are a fraction of those in the U.S. or U.K. Even medical tourism to Canada can save 30% to 60%, compared to costs in the States. Several of our close American friends have chosen to opt out of medical and dental insurance, and have traveled to Thailand or India for medical and dental care. www.bumrungrad.com

We get as much of our medical testing and treatment as possible in Chile, where a colonoscopy at a top-notch hospital costs $250, compared to $1500 to $3000 in the U.S. **Judyth:** A 25-minute IV infusion that was prescribed for me a couple of years ago cost $3500 in Seattle and $300-400 in Chile. Our dentist there is a skilled Argentine endodontist with over 30 years of experience, who practices solo in a rural home clinic with a great view of *Volcan Villarrica* from the dental chair. He charges less than 30%-50% of what we pay for comparable care in the U.S.

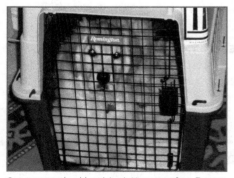

Oso, two months old, arriving in Vancouver from Toronto

TRAVELING WITH YOUR FURRY FAMILY

We travel each fall from the Pacific Northwest of the U.S. to Southern Chile with our three golden retrievers (nearly 14,000 miles round trip). Especially on long or international trips, do your research months in advance. If you wait even a month before your trip, it can be too late to meet the veterinary requirements. Fewer countries than you would think actually have quarantines, but count on strict, country-specific rules. You definitely do not want to find yourself and your pet(s) stuck between borders, or at an airport. In addition to the agricultural department requirements of the countries of origin and destination, each airline has its own regulations, which are best obtained online rather than by phone.

No Dog Left Behind

A recent Dallas-Santiago flight was highly stressful for us. Despite having made reservations for the dogs 330 days in advance, just as we were about to board the plane, the ramp supervisor informed us matter-of-factly: "I am sorry, but the combined weight of your dogs is too much for the amount of oxygen in the pet cargo hold. You will need to leave one behind. We can either fly the dog tomorrow as cargo, or one of you can postpone your trip by a day and fly with the dog tomorrow." Us: "That is unacceptable. We will not fly without all of our dogs onboard. We advised you of their size nearly a year ago, and the five of us have another connecting flight to catch tomorrow, which we would forfeit." A ten-minute standoff followed, during which all of the other passengers boarded the plane. Finally, just before the doors closed, the ramp supervisor approached us: "We rigged up a pallet for the dogs. You're good to go." We zipped onto the plane, just in time to hear: "Our departure will be delayed by thirty minutes while we accommodate the dogs on board." Any grumbles of the other passengers were drowned out by our audible sighs of relief.

Be sure to find out about:

- Are animals permitted on the airline? A close friend recently went to great lengths to rescue a Chilean street dog and, to his great relief, found an adoptive home in Los Angeles. But between his investigation and the actual flight a month later, Delta Airlines had changed their rules and no longer allowed pets on the flight.

- Cost: $100 to $200 per pet is a ballpark estimate. If you fly two different airlines from point A to point B, you could be charged twice.

- Crate type and size: Some airlines allow small pets to be carried onboard internationally and others do not. Rules about crate size can change in midstream. Last year we bought one larger crate to accommodate our taller, male golden retriever, and advised American Airlines nearly a year in advance, only to be informed upon check-in the larger crate was no longer permitted on our flight. It worked out, but barely, and had he been even an inch taller, he couldn't have flown with us.

- Temperature: Pets are not supposed to fly if the temperature of the departing city is over 85F or under about 40F. We carefully time our flights to avoid the heat of the day or the year and got our vet to write a letter saying that our dogs could fly in weather down to 32F.

- To Medicate or Not: Some airlines suggest or require tranquilizers. U.S. airlines recommend that owners not sedate their animals. Try Rescue Remedy or homeopathic *Aconite* first. One breeder, who traveled extensively with her champion Tibetan mastiffs, warned us that a tranquilized dog loses his sea legs and becomes wobbly, which is dangerous in the case of excessive turbulence. Use your own judgment—we do give our highly sensitive golden, Oso, a pre-flight Valium.

- The Ins and Outs of Food and Drink: Flying is terribly dehydrating. We plan a 4-5 hour layover, during which we give plenty of water, food, and bathroom breaks. We still find that our dogs become almost desperately thirsty. It is advised to freeze crate water bottles the night before, but ours cracked. Make sure your country of entry allows dog food: Chile does not. We place a comfy, absorbent pad covering the crate bottom, though it inevitably gets soaking wet from the dripping and shaking of the water bottle. Legally, animals are not supposed to fly more than 10 hours or so without being watered, fed, and a chance to pee or poop.

- If you need someone to pick up your beloved pet at an airport for a change of planes or other help, check out The International Pet and Animal Transport Association. A fabulous service. www.ipata.org/

PLAN TO MAKE A DIFFERENCE

In addition to enjoying meeting new friends and seeing the world, an increasing number of travelers are trying to help however they can. This can take the form of travel to promote environmental sustainability, starting an NGO (non-governmental organization) to ease suffering and spread wealth, volunteering as part of your travel experience, or staying with families and local hosts as a global citizen, rather than in hotels, hostels, or other forms of paid lodging.

Ecotourism: The Green Way to Travel

Ecotourism is based on several key principles:

- Minimize impact.

- Build environmental and cultural awareness and respect.

- Provide positive experiences for both visitors and hosts.

- Provide direct financial benefits for conservation.

- Provide financial benefits and empowerment for local people.

- Raise sensitivity to host countries' political, environmental, and social climate. www.ecotourism.org

An increasing number of environmentally-conscious tourists are dedicated to keeping the environment as pristine as possible, supporting sustainable tourism, and helping the local people and land culturally, economically and environmentally. Many of our expat friends in Chile came 20 to 30 years ago to save the Chilean temperate rainforests, *Araucaria* (monkey puzzle) and other native trees, which were being cut down for plantations of monoculture pine and eucalyptus trees for wood and toilet paper. They made a powerful and lasting impact. Another option is to choose green lodging as a way to cut, or make up for, your carbon footprint.

Voluntourism: Lending hands and hearts

Voluntourism is defined as "The conscious, seamlessly integrated combination of voluntary service to a destination and the best, traditional elements of travel — arts, culture, geography, history and 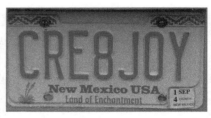 recreation — in that destination... This is travel that unites your purpose and passion, and ignites your enthusiasm." www.voluntourism.org You are sure to find a volunteer organization to suit you. The following are but a few. Homeopaths Without Borders, a nonprofit humanitarian organization established in 1996, has offered homeopathic treatment and education in Honduras, El Salvador, Guatemala, the Dominican Republic, Trinidad, Haiti, Cuba, and Sri Lanka (following the 2004 tsunami). In 2012, volunteers provided homeopathic care to nearly 900 Haitians. www.homeopathswithoutborders-na.org

Another highly worthy homeopathic avenue for voluntourism is Homoeopathy for Health in Africa, which provides free holistic treatment for people living with HIV/AIDS in Tanzania. Founded by Jeremy Sherr, an internationally respected homeopath of 30+ years, and his wife Camilla. http://www.homeopathyforhealthinafrica.org/

Countless options exist, many for young travelers, to assist in community projects abroad. Some of our patients and their families travel regularly to Latin America to build schools and stock libraries. Two of our Canadian friends, one a homeopath, started an amazing Children's Village in Guatemala with rich opportunities for adult and student voluntourists. We are profoundly inspired by their efforts to create *Project Somos*. www.projectsomos.org

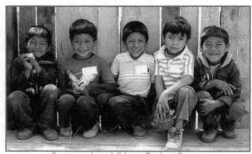
Guatemalan children, Project Somos

One friend who was born in the Dominican Republic, educated in the U.S., then lived for a number of years on Whidbey Island, Washington, where we met, founded a Sister Island program to give back, in a big way, by starting a school and medical clinic in the village of *Cruz Verde* where she grew up. www.sisterislandproject.org

An extraordinarily successful, green eco-volunteer organization is WWOOF (World Wide Opportunities on Organic Farms). It is a work-share scheme for organic farms where work is ex-changed for accommodation and meals. The "wwoofers" get to work the land, breathe fresh air, contrib-ute to greening the planet, and provide willing hands for farmers who could never manage all the responsibilities themselves. Plus a comfy bed, good company, and they get to be "hands on" in the kitchen to prepare the healthy, organic food they helped to grow! www.wwoof.org

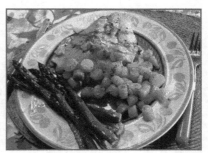

Wild Alaskan salmon with organic baby carrots and asparagus

A Fascinating Favela

In February of 2010, we rented out our Chilean home to a gringo tourist and headed off to Brazil for a month, planning to rendezvous with friends for a few days before returning to the U.S. Upon landing at the Rio airport, the LAN gate agent, highly distraught, advised us, "There has been a massive earthquake in Chile and the world is ending." Alaska Airlines got us on a free-miles flight to Seattle the next day, and we found a lovely hostel in artsy Santa Teresa. Consulting Trip Advisor, were intrigued by the notion of a *favela* (slum) tour.

Our 4-hour tour of Rocinha, considered to be the largest

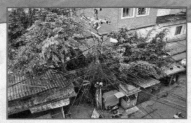

Illegal electrical wire hookup Rocinha favela, Rio de Janeiro, Brazil

slum in the Americas, was one of the most unique sightseeing experiences of our lives. Arriving at our drop-off point in a group bus, each of us hopped on the back of a motorcycle with a Brazilian biker, and zoomed up a steep hill to the slum. Not a moment to think about helmets; we were just holding on for dear life! That was the least of the potential danger, as we learned in the briefing that followed. We were to take NO photos of anyone visibly chatting on a cell phone, as they might be armed drug dealers who wouldn't appreciate being exposed on Facebook! The tour, organized by a non-profit social work organization functioned through the good graces of the Rocinha drug lords, as long as the rules were followed. During our up-close and personal walk through the narrow back lanes of the *favela*, we had to step carefully because of broken pavement, garbage, shit, and various and sundry cats and dogs. The approximately 200,000 mostly destitute residents haphazardly connected thousands of wires to the electric cables, creating a maze of wiring, none of which was metered. The same was done with cable TV wiring. The graffiti art gallery, hosted by the talented young artists, was a treat. The dwellings in the *favelas* were stacked vertically, and the residents allowed to sell the air space above so that another family could build a shack above theirs.

Several years later, as part of a pre-Olympics cleanup sweep by the Brazilian police and army, the drug lords in Rocinha were ousted, and enough ammunition found to arm a small country. www.cristotours.com/2012/07/favela-tour.html

Gift As You Go

Short of volunteering, there are innumerable small ways to share as you travel. The smallest gift, which you take for granted, can open a heart and bridge a cultural chasm. Some travelers take postcards or small calendars. Sweet treats are popular, but there

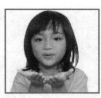

are healthier and more teeth-friendly options. Go to a local dollar store and load up on small, light, cheap goodies to share. Even pens! Take a special gift to your host family—a traditional item from home is a great reminder of the lovely time you shared. You don't have to gift materially. Gift yourself: a lovely smile, a heartfelt greeting, a shared glance. Graciously open a door or help an elderly or handicapped person cross the road. Share a song, a dance or photo. These trinkets and moments can be unforgettable.

Dive Into a Different Culture

There are more culturally experiential alternatives to sightseeing, staying in hotels, hostels, vacation rentals, or couch surfing. www.couchsurfing.org/ On "The Other Tour", an alternative, socially conscious tour of Istanbul, the exuberant school children delighted in seeing their photos that we had just snapped. Their giggles were more memorable than any tourist sites or monuments.

We are members of a worldwide, cross-cultural peace program called SERVAS. Particularly popular in Europe, it allows travelers to either host or stay with a local family, for the purpose of promoting understanding and cultural exchange among like-minded individuals and families in most countries of the world. It is an excellent way to be a tourist in a more intimate way and to expand your family of friends. We spent a week with a gracious and hospitable Argentine artist in Buenos Aires and made other good friends, who later stayed with us in our home in Chile.

Travel Smart: Work the Web to Be a Savvy Traveler

The internet has revolutionized travel planning and research, but experienced travelers that we are, we still have a lot to learn to get the most out of the digital info out there on the web. Here are some picks of our own and some by the N.Y. Times columnist Seth Kugel, the Frugal Traveler: http://tinyurl.com/frugal-traveler-picks

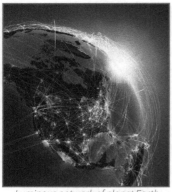

Luminous network of planet Earth

TRAVEL PLANNING AND REVIEWS
Trip Advisor
The most well-known combination of traveler lodging reviews, comments, and photos of hotels, activities and locations. Well liked and respected by millions of travelers. Owned by Expedia. com, it rates lodging, restaurants, and sights worldwide, as well as connecting you with booking sites. www.tripadvisor.com

Virtual Tourist
Also owned by Expedia. A less commercial community of travelers posting lodging, location and activity reviews and photos. Worth a look. More community-oriented than Trip Advisor, but not as popular. Virtual Tourists actually stage get-togethers for members. Several million VT readers recently voted Torres del Paine Park in Chilean Patagonia the "Eighth Wonder of the World!" www.virtualtourist.com

Expat Blogs
Blogs from expatriates living in various parts of the world, sharing their travel and cultural experiences of the country they have adopted. Their tips on how to blend in with the locals or adjust and adapt to the way things are done there can be invaluable if you are going to spend more than a few days in a particular country. Fascinating insights abound in these blogs. www.expatsblog.com/blogs

Stay
Prepares a social-media-connected city guide to hotels, restaurants and activities that you can access off-line on your mobile device during your trip. Share your city guide with family and friends, off-line saving roaming charges. www.stay.com

MatadorNetwork

A fascinating site filled with cultural blog excerpts and photos from travelers all over the world, who form an online community. We found an account of the fire-breathing *curanderos* in Iluman, Ecuador, that mirrored our own experience. www.matadornetwork.com

Skypicker

Helps you figure out where you can fly within your budget, only in Europe, and only on very cheap flights. You need your approximate departure date and how many days you will be staying, and you get a list of the cheapest flights to and from your destination. www.skypicker.com

Seat61

According to the Frugal Traveler, the "Man in Seat 61", Mark Smith, is the expert on European train rides, and can get you the right ride at the best price. www.seat61.com

GETTING THERE AND STAYING THERE
Kayak

A well-known mega search engine for finding some of the least expensive airfares, flight combinations and hotel bookings across the web. Easy to use. Kayak searches your request and refers you to the airline, hotel, or car rental to book. Our favorite flight site. Combines searching the big three with many lesser sites for a complete picture of your flight or hotel options. www.kayak.com

Best Travel Coupon

Powerful search engine which claims access to the most hotels of any travel site and to post the lowest prices for hotels and airfares. Their motto is: "We search hundreds of sites. You get the best price." Click on "Proven Results" to see the differences. www.besttravelcoupon.com

Vayama

Specializes in international flights and offers "the best selection of international travel deals." Their search includes 500 airlines worldwide for a good selection and a best price guarantee. We used them to book a low-cost flight to Brazil on GOL Airlines, a carrier that was unknown to us at the time. www.vayama.com

Trivago
Worldwide hotel search engine with 151 booking sites and 638,713 hotels and counting. It can turn up hotels that are overlooked on other booking sites. It also has a member/community aspect where each action you do to support the community, such as writing a review or uploading a photo generates a small commission. www.trivago.com

Hotels
An excellent booking service that allows multiple filters to find the kind of hotel you want at the price you want in the place you want. Doesn't compare across other booking sites. Good customer service. May not be the lowest prices, but has very good last minute deals. www.hotels.com

Booking
Extremely easy-to-use booking service with great reviews from customers. Offers discounted prices. Customer service is a plus. You don't have to pay the reservation until you check in. Has a 24-hour best-price guarantee. www.booking.com

Priceline
William Shatner, the Priceline Negotiator, has been the spokesman for this somewhat unconventional booking agency until 2012. The old Captain Kirk exhorts, in his dying scene for Priceline (before the bus plunges from a bridge in Asia, killing off his character): "Save yourselves—Save money!" That's what Priceline has been doing online since 1998. As long as you don't mind not knowing exactly where you are staying, or how the airlines are going to get you there, or which rental car company you are renting from. You just name your own price for a blind reservation that won't be revealed until you've paid up. Great deals for flexible travelers with time on their hands, whose first priority is saving money rather than being certain about travel plans. www.priceline.com

Airbnb.com
This site describes itself as "a community marketplace for unique spaces", and has the photos to prove it. Choose from over 192 countries and 33,000 cities; anything from a room to a mansion that the owner is offering. Room with the host or have the place to yourself for a stated price. www.airbnb.com

VRBO and HomeAway

Great if you want to rent a home or apartment for 3 days to 3 months or more. Highly reputable site, with great variety of homes. Worth checking out whether your group is 2 or 10. www.vrbo.com, www.homeaway.com

OTHER USEFUL SITES
Seat Guru

A service of Trip Advisor, Seat Guru will show you the seating map of your flight, with in-depth comments about seats with limited recline, reduced legroom and misaligned windows. Be comfortable with the knowledge that your seat will be comfortable, too, at least as far as airline seats go. www.seatguru.com

Yapta

Track changes in your airfare after you have paid, so you can apply for a credit or voucher if it goes down significantly. www.yapta.com

Bing Travel

Search for airfares and use the Price Predictor to determine whether you should buy now or later. www.bingtravel.com

Expert Flyer

Be an email message away from finding your favorite plane seat. This nifty site offers free seat alerts and, for a minimal monthly fee, handy info on flight availability, seats, fares, and how to best use your miles. www.expert-flyer.com

What to Take With You on Your Journey

TRAVEL DOCS AND I.D.

If you take only one thing, let it be your passport, with any visas stamped inside. (Or, better yet, take the Savvy Travel Docs—send us tickets!) You can get money in most places from an ATM and can have credit cards sent or wired, but losing your passport can drastically alter your plans.

If you travel extensively, be sure your passport has plenty of blank pages for visas. Take note of the expiration date—some countries (such as Israel) refuse entry unless there are six months left on the passport. A rabbi friend, on his way to lead a tour in Israel, was turned back and missed his trip!

CASH AND CARDS

- Limit cash. ATMs are widely available and you have less to lose in case of theft. Cash can also be bulky. Once in India we exchanged $500 for rupees and were given four stacks of small-denomination bills that took up about 6" of space! "Very sorry, *memsaab*, that's all we have." When we do get trip cash at our bank in the U.S., we inspect each bill, front, and back, for writing or tears. If not perfect, they may be rejected. Once we were stuck with four out of eight of our $100 bills.

- In some places, such as Buenos Aires, small change is guarded like gold. Obtaining coins for a bus is next to impossible. Better to know ahead.

- Count on transaction fees for cash withdrawals. Take out what you need for a week rather than for a day, as fees per transaction can be up to eight dollars or more.

- On holidays, or for other reasons, cash machines may run out of money.

- We prefer to use ATMs where you slide your card in and out, rather than one that swallows your card, then spits it out at the end of the transaction. These machines have swallowed a card or two, much to our dismay. One Australian adventurer used this kind of ATM in Paraguay on a Friday. Her card was similarly devoured. The next Monday she discovered that her checking account had been completely emptied.

- Be careful frequenting cash machines in dicey areas, especially at night.

- If traveling for months at a time, be aware of the expiration dates on your credit cards and plan to have the new ones sent to you.

- Use a secure, encrypted method to carry passwords. Avoid e-mailing passwords, credit card expiration dates, and other financial or

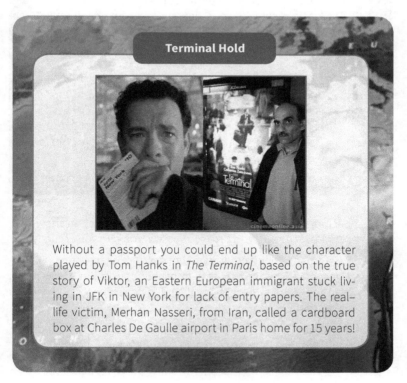

Terminal Hold

Without a passport you could end up like the character played by Tom Hanks in *The Terminal*, based on the true story of Viktor, an Eastern European immigrant stuck living in JFK in New York for lack of entry papers. The real–life victim, Merhan Nasseri, from Iran, called a cardboard box at Charles De Gaulle airport in Paris home for 15 years!

Dubbed "Sir Alfred" by the airport employees, despite earning six-figure money from the movie rights, and ultimately legalizing his documents, he became too introverted and mistrustful of people outside to live anywhere but the airport. The fame and movie income were used to purchase only a second set of clothes and some books. Take with you in a handy spot:

1. A copy of all electronic tickets, reservation confirmations, and important tour or travel communication. Although an online airline confirmation is usually adequate, there are times when flights are abruptly changed or canceled, and you need your locator number in hand. It is often not possible to access this information online due to lack of WIFI at the ticket counter. Save the boarding passes, too, in case you need to claim your frequent flyer miles later.

2. A document with your itinerary and contact information can be invaluable, especially for long and complicated trips.

3. One or two copies of credit cards, driver's license, passport I.D. page, debit cards stashed separately from your wallet or money belt. Leave all cards that you don't need at home. Don't invest in an international driver's license without checking first to make sure you need it. They only last a year and a driver's license from home is often adequate.

personal information, especially in cyber cafes. Get an encrypted, cloud-based service to take your passwords with you securely.

- Save money using a credit card that does not charge additional foreign fees. Advise the issuing bank of your travel plans. Even so, you may find your card blocked by the fraud department, requiring you to call them.

- Make sure your money belt is the right size for you and your valuables, comfortable, and accessible. We take one for the waist and another around the neck, depending on what we're wearing.

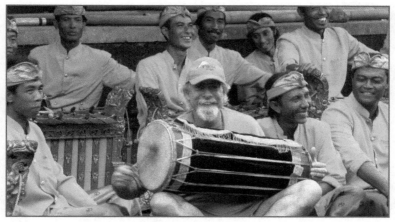

Bob drumming in Bali with new friends

DON'T LEAVE HOME WITHOUT THIS BOOK AND A HOMEOPATHIC TRAVEL KIT

Be sure to take this book, either in paper, Kindle, or other e-book form. What you save on a few ounces cannot compare to having at your fingertips a wealth of useful information that you can use for yourself, your family, and those whom you meet on the road. Call it being a global Good Samaritan. A photographer patient who travels to the ends of the earth snapping takes our kit hither and yon. In Peru he ended up being the group doctor!

There are various potencies (strengths) of homeopathic medicines, ranging from low (6X or 12X) to average (30C, the most common for acute illnesses and what we include in our kits) to high (200C, 1M, 10M, the higher potencies). Basically, the lower the potency, the more often you need to take it. What is most important is to find the medicine that is the best match for the symptoms. The potency is secondary. You will typically have to take a 6X or 12X potency every couple of hours, a 30C potency at most three times a day, and a 200C or 1M potency only once, or a couple of times, during the illness. We will refer to 30C potencies in the rest of this section, since that is what you will most likely be using. You can also find combination homeopathic medicines, including several different medicines, for particular conditions. These are an option, if they are all you can find, but, if a single medicine best fits the symptoms, take it.

HOMEOPATHIC SELF-CARE MEDICINE KIT

★ Our top pick if you are traveling down the block or around the
world. This sturdy, lightweight, yellow plastic kit contains the 50 most
common medicines for first aid
and acute conditions. It is a companion to our larger book, *Homeopathic Self-Care: The Quick and Easy*

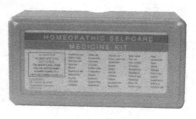

Guide for the Whole Family. (30C potency, 5 1/2" long x 3" wide x 1 3/4"
high; one-pound.) An ideal kit if you want 50 rather than 36 remedies. The
pellets are tiny, so the quantity is enough for years, if not for life. **We have sold
over two thousand of these popular kits over the past 17 years.** Refills are
easily available from Washington Homeopathic Products.
Order this kit from www.healthyhomeopathy.com/shop

Aconite	Gelsemium	Podophyllum
Allium cepa	Glonoine	Pulsatilla
Argentum nitricum	Hepar sulph	Rhus tox
Apis	Hypericum	Rumex
Arnica	Ignatia	Ruta
Arsenicum album	Ipecac	Sarsaparilla
Belladonna	Kali bichromicum	Sepia
Bryonia	Lachesis	Silica
Carbo veg	Ledum	Spongia tosta
Chamomilla	Lycopodium	Staphysagria
China	Magnesia phos	Sulphur
Cocculus	Mercurius	Symphytum
Coffea	Natrum mur	Tabacum
Colocynthis	Nux vomica	Urtica urens
Drosera	Petroleum	Veratrum album
Euphrasia	Phosphorus	
Ferrum phos	Phytolacca	

36 HOMEOPATHIC REMEDY TRAVEL KIT

★ **This is our recommendation if you want a smaller, lighter kit with fourteen fewer, and slightly different, remedies.** A convenient, affordable, robust kit that also makes an excellent companion to this book. The kit includes one or more medicines for

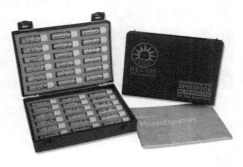

each of the health problems in our book. It comes in a green, plastic case measuring 5.6" long x 4.4" wide x 1.5" high and weighs 10.6 oz. About 35 pillules per glass bottle. You can also order this kit from www.healthyhomeopathy.com/shop.

The following 30C-potency medicines are included:

Aconite	Chelidonium	Manganum
Apis	China	Mercurius
Argentum nitricum	Cocculus	Natrum muriaticum
Arnica	Cuprum	Nux vomica
Arsenicum album	Eupatorium perf.	Podophyllum
Belladonna	Gelsemium	Pulsatilla
Bellis perennis	Hepar sulph	Rhus tox
Bryonia	Hypericum	Ruta
Camphora	Ignatia	Silica
Cantharis	Ipecac	Staphysagria
Carbo veg	Lathyrus	Urtica
Chamomilla	Ledum	Veratrum

Regardless of which kit you choose, you can purchase additional medicines, at any time, for your specific needs.

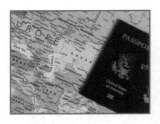

BUYING HOMEOPATHIC MEDICINES ON THE ROAD

You may be able to find what you need during your travels, though taking a kit is a much better plan. Homeopathic medicines are available in the U.S., Europe, India, Mexico, Argentina, Brazil, Australia, New Zealand, Kenya, and Israel.

Depending on the country:

U.S.

- Health food stores or natural food supermarket, co-op
- U.S. pharmacies (Pharmaca, Walgreens, Rite-Aid, or CVS)
- Hahnemann Labs in California. www.hahnemannlabs.com
- You can order a kit from our website. www.healthyhomeopathy.com

Canada

In most pharmacies, health food stores, homeopathic pharmacies.

U.K.

Homeopathic pharmacies, health food stores, regular pharmacies.

- Helios Homeopathic Pharmacy www.helios.co.uk

Western Europe

Most pharmacies in France, but not in potencies above 30C. Widely available in Germany, Holland, and Scandinavia. In health food stores in larger cities in Spain and Portugal as well as homeopathic pharmacies.

Central and South America

Homeopathic pharmacies and sometimes in regular pharmacies, especially major cities. Widely available in Argentina. May need a doctor's prescription in Brazil.

Australia and New Zealand
Health food stores, pharmacies, homeopathic pharmacies, homeopaths.

Russia
From homeopaths in large cities.

India
Prevalent in pharmacies and homeopathic clinics throughout India, Sri Lanka, Bangladesh.

Africa
Homeopaths and pharmacies in South Africa. May be difficult elsewhere.

Homeopathic pharmacies that ship internationally:

- Helios Homeopathic Pharmacy www.helios.co.uk

- Boiron homeopathic medicines are widely distributed throughout Europe and the U.S., and many countries worldwide. www.boiron.com

- Homeopathy World ships a variety of kits throughout the world. www.homeopathyworld.com

Check online to see if homeopathic medicines are readily available in the country to which you are traveling.

BASIC FIRST AID KIT

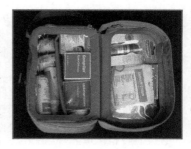

In addition to your homeopathic kit, it is a good idea to take a kit with basic first aid supplies, especially if you will be away from pharmacies. They are widely available in various sizes, weights, and contents. If you make your own, consult existing kits for ideas of what to include. With a homeopathic kit and the recommendations from this book, you should be able to take fewer pharmaceutical medications with you. You can find a variety of excellent kits to suit your needs at Recreational Equipment (REI). www.rei.com

HERBS AND NUTRITIONAL SUPPLEMENTS

There are a couple of items that we recommend for all travelers, regardless of destination or the nature of the trip.

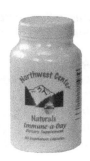

- **Immune Support**—Our favorites are Immune-a-Day and Olive Leaf Relief! These are private-labeled supplements that we sell through our clinic. www.healthyhomeopathy.com/shop

- Another option is EHB (Integrative Therapeutics). We have used these immune-boosting products successfully for many years. Or choose your own. The key is to have them handy enough that you can start taking them four times a day at the very first sign of a cold, sore throat, or flu. This practice has saved us from catching a cold many times over the years.

- **Calendula** (marigold) cream—This is our mainstay for cuts, scrapes, rashes, and sunburn. **Judyth:** I became convinced of its amazing healing powers while working in a free tent clinic in Old Delhi (1981). Our only tools were soap and *Calendula*, even for deep, infected gashes. This simple flower worked miracles. Another alternative is colloidal silver.

FOOD EN ROUTE

In the frenzy of packing, remember to take healthy snacks. Don't get caught starving on a red eye or overnight bus, paying a fortune for the simplest and least nutritious food in an airport, or being forced to eat unhygienic fare that may land you in the loo. Take sliced veggies and healthy dip, bread and cheese, protein bars, and a couple of hard boiled eggs. Pack fresh fruit and veggies ahead of time to insure that they are pesticide-free, or that you can wash it in water you trust.

Judyth: I watched in Israel as the vendor liberally sprayed Raid on his produce. Give me a fly in my soup any day! Check customs regulations first to make sure you can enter with your stash. Undeclared fruits, vegetables, dairy and meat products can result in a hefty fine in countries with strict agricultural regulations. We were busted in Chile to the tune of $70 for a package of undeclared dried cranberries for a Thanksgiving feast. It was a bad morning for a couple of other young women, as well, thanks to an overly conscientious customs agent. One was fined for peppercorns and the other popcorn! Now we know to *always* declare *something*. Then we don't get dinged, even if they make us toss the item.

Be sure you know which health prevention items you can take on the plane and which you can't. During a week-long kayak trip to Prince William Sound in Alaska, after hearing a gruesome grizzly tale in Cordova, we bought pepper spray to ward off grizzlies. We had originally promised ourselves to only go with guides carrying guns, but that was

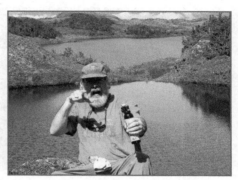
Bob practicing spraying a grizzly

not the case. To our dismay, the spray was confiscated on our Cordova-Anchorage flight en route to Valdez. The night we pitched our tents, one large black bear ambled by not too far from our campsite. And we did spot bear scat near the icebergs, as well as a cute cub on the shore. But all ended well and bear-free.

PACK LIGHT TIPS
Traveling well is not having to trudge around, miserable, and running the risk of wrenching your back. Be a smart, light packer.

- Know your carry-on and checked baggage allowances. Cheap, lightweight luggage scales, available in airports, can save you pricey excess baggage fees.

- Find just the right luggage for your needs. The vast array of lightweight, attractive, wheeling and/or backpack combos is dazzling. We swear by our Eagle Creek wheeling packs, though lighter versions are now available. When we were limited to 20 pounds on an island hopper within the Galapagos, we used our 18-ounce Gossamer Gear ultra-light backpacks. www.gossamergear.com

- Travel guru Rick Steves (*Europe Through The Back Door*) shepherds tens of thousands of travelers, of all ages and travel styles, through Europe. They allow one carry-on bag. Period. A patient recently returned from one of these speedy jaunts to Italy, and described how miserable a couple of the participants were dragging their ridiculously heavy bags onto buses and down cobblestone streets. Better a carefree trip than a hernia. www.ricksteves.com

- You need very few clothes when traveling—just a few mix-and-match, comfy, easy-to-wash, versatile outfits, some underwear, and scarves or jewelry to dress up. Plus your sportswear and gear and a bathing suit. No one will care how boring your wardrobe may be.

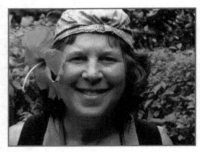

Flower child. Galapagos Islands, Ecuador

- Be aware of cultural mores and sensitivity regarding dress, head coverings, bathing wear, sleeve and dress length. When traveling in Islamic areas, tuck a head scarf in your pocket for mosque visits.

- You can buy very lightweight, crinkly (no-iron), fun clothing—even sun- and bug-protected. We are loyal shoppers of REI—Recreational Equipment, Inc. REI stands by their products and happily returns any damaged items, even years later! Once they remedied a damaged tent pole by giving us a brand new tent! www.rei.com

- Enjoy a fun splurge at TravelSmith or Ex Officio. www.travelsmith.com, www.exofficio.com

- Shoes can make or break a trip. We wear our hiking boots on the plane, since they're too big and heavy to pack. Take broken-in walking shoes.

TRICKS OF THE TRAVEL-WELL TRADE

- Wet wipes—They are light, compact, and can be a breath of fresh air on red eyes, trips with multi-connecting flights, or overnight bus rides, or when you can't get a shower for two or three days. They're handy when there are no paper towels in the bathroom, or for kayak or hiking trips when fresh water is limited or unavailable.

- Mini toiletries—Perfect when every ounce or inch counts.

- Extra zip-close strong, plastic bags of various sizes. If you know you will buy fragile souvenirs, take bubble wrap.

- Since we travel with boxes to Chile, which are opened by TSA for inspection, we take a roll of strapping tape to seal them en route.

- A compact LED flashlight or headlamp if you need your hands free.

- A sarong—Use as a dress, a swim cover-up, a lightweight wrap, a sun block, a privacy or light screen, to lay on the ground for a picnic or to protect you from bugs, a shawl, or a head covering. One size fits all.

- Laundry—Take a flat, round universal sink plug, a light, plastic scrubber, and biodegradable liquid soap, so you can do laundry anytime anywhere.

- Sleep aids—A compact, neck-friendly travel pillow (we prefer buck-wheat or memory foam-filled). Polar guard booties to keep your toes toasty on a cold flight. A soft eyeshade. Comfy, effective, ear-plugs for a noisy neighbor and snorer prevention. (Don't even think of putting them in his nostrils!)

- Cotton or silk sleep sacks to save washing linens and for hygiene.

- iPod, or iPad, iPhone or Android smart phone for entertainment, phone service and to have access to apps and a GPS. Get a GSM phone for use in most countries in the world.

- Rent or buy a cheap cell phone or pre-paid chip at the airport on entry.

- Electric plugs and adaptors suitable to your travel needs.

- If you are going somewhere without clean water, small, lightweight, pen-sized UV filters are available. Make sure the battery works!

- Extra ear jacks in case they charge for them on the plane.

- We have extremely basic, light, little backpacks that weigh nothing and can be used in a pinch for water, a light lunch, and a sweater.

- We take our Australian Cool Snake necktie coolers, feather-light neck wraps filled with water-absorbing crystals to stay cool in extremely hot, dry weather. www.coolhats. com.au/cool_snakes.html

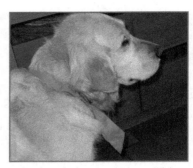

Dulce de Leche beating the heat with her Cool Snake

- A tiny, battery-operated fan is great in hot, humid, or smoky rooms.

- Locks—In addition to your luggage locks, if you travel alone and may be sleeping in an airport or need to leave your bag, pack a strong cable to tie around public seats. A padlock, with key or lock, is useful if you are staying in lodging without locking doors or with questionable security.

- Keep bag tags current, with info that makes it easy to reach you quickly—email address and phone numbers coming and going.

- If we plan to do any serious shopping, we take a nylon bag which folds or stuffs down to nothing.

- A mini sewing kit is a godsend when your pants rip down the rear!

- A mini eyeglass repair kit.

- A Swiss army knife in your checked luggage.

- If you're the adventurous type, a small role of duct tape never hurts. Once we fixed our broken tent pole with duct tape and saved our trip!

How to Stay Healthy and Safe While Traveling

SUN SAFE

The Environmental Working Group (EWG) reported that nearly half of the 500 most popular sunscreens might actually increase skin cancer risk. Only 39 of the 500 products they examined in 2010 were considered safe and effective. Apparently, in the U.S., the FDA had been aware of the potential danger for as long as a decade, without alerting the public. The main danger was due to oxybenzone, a hormone-disrupting chemical, which penetrates the skin and enters the bloodstream. Also in question were overstated claims of performance. One-fourth of the sunscreens studied in 2012 contained retinyl palmitate, a form of Vitamin A. The EWG discourages the use of these products and are pressing manufacturers to eliminate it from their sunscreens. www.ewg.org

Another concern was the use, in the U.S., of nano-sized titanium dioxide, which may have significant health implications. In addition, SPF ratings are often misleading and meaningless, offering a false sense of security resulting in users staying out in the sun longer than they should. Many sun worshippers apply much less that the recommended amount of sunscreen, resulting in a true SPF of 2 instead of what they believe to be 100. This is alarming for adults, and even more so for babies and small children.
What to do:

- Wear sun-blocking hats and clothing.
- Limit time in the sun.
- Don't be misled by claims of super-high SPF until laws change in the U.S.
- Buy a sunscreen marketed for kids, because they are less likely to contain oxybenzone and fragrances. Still read the ingredients to make your own comparison since there is hype.

- Choose sun-block sunscreens, containing zinc oxide and titanium dioxide. They offer the best UV protection without hormonal disruption.

- Lip balms are even more questionable, offering less UV protection and containing Vitamin A.

- Check the EWG site for the most up-to-date sunscreen safety research.

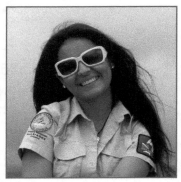

Our beautiful Galapagos National Park guide

BUGS BE GONE

Your likelihood of developing serious problems from a mosquito bite depends primarily on when, where, for how long, and in which season you are traveling. Global warming is causing tropical diseases to spread to non-tropical areas. Mosquitoes are tough to ignore and hard to love.

What are your options? First you need to decide whether bug bites are just a potential annoyance or whether you are at serious risk of joining the legions of malaria sufferers. You may even want to plan your trip accordingly, especially if you have kids, are elderly, are very insect-bite-prone, or are immune-compromised. You can opt for a safari in South Africa, for example, instead Kenya or Tanzania. Explore your options. New products are being developed all the time.

In addition to your repellant of choice, start with the other common-sense precautions: long pants and shirts, mosquito netting over beds and on hats, avoid standing, swampy water, and try not to travel during high-mosquito seasons, and stay inside at dusk. That said, read on:

- DEET: This yellowish oil is the most common ingredient in insect repellants and protects against mosquitoes, ticks, chiggers, and other insects. Developed by the U.S. Army after the jungle combat of World War II, it was originally tested as a pesticide on farm fields. The U.S. began using it in 1946 and the public in 1957. It was heavily used during the Vietnam War. It seems that both genders of mosquito intensely dislike the smell of DEET, as well as that of that of other repellants such as eucalyptol, linalool, and thujone (homeopaths will recognize this as a cedar derivative from the homeopathic medicine *Thuja*). DEET is sold as a spray or lotion in concentrations up to 100%. The higher the concentration, the longer the action. Formulations containing 100% DEET offer 12 hours of protection, and those with 20%-34% offer 3-6 hours.

- DEET has been found to inhibit central nervous system activity in insects and in mammals. Manufacturers recommend limiting use to exposed areas and clothing rather than underneath, and washing off the product when no longer needed. Minor symptoms include insomnia, mood changes, and impaired thinking. More serious symptoms, though rare, include seizures and death. The *American Academy of Pediatrics* approves the use of DEET for children older than two months. Health Canada banned the sale of 30%+ DEET preparations, recommended 10% or less strength for children under two, and also limited number of daily applications.

- Permethrin: A synthetic chemical, it kills ticks and prevents mosquito-borne diseases including dengue fever and malaria. It is most commonly sprayed over outer clothing, and is used to treat mosquito nets. It is apparently 2,250 times more toxic to ticks than to humans, and only 1% of the active ingredient is absorbed into the body if applied to the skin. We used the spray method successfully during a week-long kayaking trip in Southern Alaska. A large netted tent for cooking was invaluable. www.tickencounter.org/prevention/permethrin

- Lemon Eucalyptus: Made from the gum tree, the main essential oil, *Citronella*, has become a popular additive to natural bug repellants. It may interfere with single-dose homeopathic medicines.

STASH YOUR STUFF
Your safety and your life are far more important than any possessions. Give thieves whatever they want in order to avoid injury. Use a money belt,

especially on crowded streets, markets (a haven for professional pickpockets), and airports. Hold on tightly to purses and conceal cameras. Don't display wads of cash in public places, keep your jewelry simple, and be alert for people behaving suspiciously around cash machines. Keep a credit or debit card in a place other than your wallet or purse or stash some cash in an unlikely place, so you always have a reserve. Some couples carry credit cards from different accounts or banks, in case one is blocked or stolen. Other travelers carry a decoy wallet with just a few bills to offer up in a worst-case scenario, while holding onto their hidden money belt. Most muggers are after cash, cameras, and electronics that can be easily fenced.

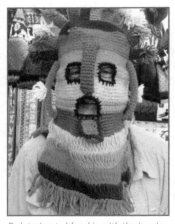

A retired Canadian couple was innocently strolling down a busy Santiago street in broad daylight. A thief ripped the purse from her arm and the camera that hung around his neck. A policeman happened by just at that moment. The man and the cop set off in hot pursuit. After a block, the desperate thief tossed both stolen items in the air. They landed on the ground, but were salvageable. The couple ended up with a slightly damaged camera, some bruises, and a tale to tell their grandkids.

Bob trying to blend in with the locals

Keep your luggage in sight, locked, and with the strap around a part of your body. Take luggage locks and a combination padlock on your trip, and use them. Do not leave your luggage unattended. Make sure your hotel room is safe before leaving valuables behind, or use the designated room safe or the front desk. A spare padlock can be useful if you need to lock a room that has no door lock. Be particularly careful about expensive electronic devices such as cameras, smart phones, iPads, and computers. They can be easily lifted from a pocket, seat, or rental car. And be sure to back up any documents you can't afford to lose!

Traveling on a familiar bus in Chile, on our way to *Torres del Paine* National

Park and to Argentine Patagonia, lulled us into a false sense of security. Both foggy with head colds, we were oblivious to having stashed our camera and money belts in a daypack on the shelf above us. A quick-as-a-flash, nimble-fingered thief ripped us off when we were resting, made off with $500 cash, our camera and passports. The passports were soon recovered, thanks to a police report that alerted the U.S. Embassy. But it was a hassle that could have been avoided by just remembering that money belts are to be worn!

EAT WELL

What to eat and what to avoid? When is street food safe? What if you are graciously invited to eat at someone's home? You can enjoy all of these experiences with a few essential guidelines. The biggest sources of unsafe food are dirty hands, flies and contaminated water. You won't always be able to avoid con-tamination, especially when invited to eat by local or indig-enous hosts.

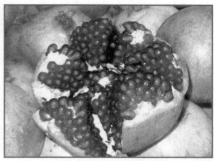

De-seeding pomegranates made simple: https://www.youtube.com/watch?v=aUsfw-KppCU

Some simple guidelines:

- "Wash it, peel it, boil it, or forget it," is an adage that holds water. The safest food is fresh, well cooked, baked, broiled, boiled or deep-fried.

- Avoid salad bars unless you are in a country with a very safe tap water supply, or you are frequenting a tourist-friendly restaurant that knows to wash raw vegetables carefully. Choose cooked vegetables instead.

- Peel or wash fruits well with a fruit and vegetable wash or mild detergent.

- Avoid eating at food stalls or restaurants where the dishes and utensils are poorly washed in cold water. Avoid food handled by others with uncertain hygiene.

- Avoid GMO (genetically-modified) food when possible.

- Spicy food is not necessarily safer, and may give you the runs.

- Watch out for unrefrigerated dairy products unless they are pasteurized or freshly cultured. If you are staying at a farm with reliable hygiene, raw dairy might be fine. We make delicious, unpasteurized yogurt, soft cheese, and ice cream from our dairy sheep milk in Chile.

- Shellfish and prawns may grow in contaminated waters, carry neurological shellfish poisons like red tide, and transmit disease if not well-cooked. Raw meat and fish (sushi, *ceviche*) can make you sick if not carefully prepared.

BOIL OR PURIFY YOUR BEVERAGES

Drink only bottled, filtered or boiled water and beverages! Never drink tap water or brush your teeth with it unless you are sure it's safe. Boil or purify water or un-bottled beverages to make them safer to drink. Waterborne illness is highly prevalent in the developing world, including parasites such as worms and flukes that can infect the intestines and liver, and protozoa, and *Giardia lamblia, Entamoeba histolytica,* and *Cryptosporidium parva*, which can cause severe and chronic diarrhea. Many types of bacteria are waterborne and can cause cholera, typhoid, salmonella and other forms of traveler's diarrhea. Viruses that cause hepatitis A and polio are also transmitted by water.

Follow these simple guidelines:

- Boil! Your best chance to kill offending organisms is death by boiling. Boil longer at higher altitudes as the boiling temperature decreases by 1 degree C per every 300 meters of altitude.

- Filter! You can remove most bacteria, but not viruses, with a fine filter, ceramic filters being the best, and the pores should be no larger than 0.5 microns. Pre-filtering might be necessary if the water is dirty. Activated charcoal filters are good for removing chemicals and chlorine, but do nothing for bacteria or viruses.

- UV light purifiers such as the small, light SteriPEN are 99.9% effective against bacteria, viruses, and protozoa. Immerse for 48 sec-

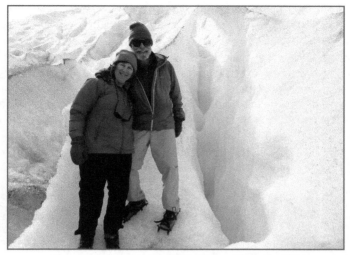

Enjoying pure water on the Perito Moreno Glacier, Argentina

onds for half a liter and 96 seconds for a liter. They do not eliminate chemicals or dirt in the water.

- Better drinking through chemistry—silver, chlorine and iodine are used to purify drinking water.

- Colloidal silver is harmless and tasteless, but slow-acting, and not useful against Giardia or amoebas.

- Chlorine takes 10-30 minutes, is harmless and effective when used correctly. Again Giardia and amoebas are best removed by filtration or by long exposure to chlorine. Iodine is quick and effective in 10 minutes, and kills cysts more quickly than chlorine. Both chlorine and iodine can affect the taste of the water to the point of being undrinkable. Buffered Vitamin C tablets can help offset the unpleasant taste of the iodine. Iodine should not be used by people with thyroid problems or by pregnant women, or should at least be removed after purification by a carbon filter.

- A rule of thumb: Filter first, purify second.

IF YOU DO GET SICK IN A FOREIGN COUNTRY

Medical care varies widely throughout the world. In the developed countries such as in Europe, the U.S., Japan, Australia and New Zealand, parts of South America, and in major cities in the developing world, you can easily find private doctors, clinics, and hospitals offering conventional inpatient medical care. In rural areas, hospitals and clinics are less available or non-existent, or have relatively primitive facilities and standards of hygiene. Local customs for receiving medical care vary. In India, for example, you can find modern medical and homeopathic care available in private and government hospitals, but, in many hospitals, you will need to provide your own food, bedding, medicines and bandages.

For these reasons, we recommend good medical insurance that covers foreign emergencies, or travel insurance with medical and evacuation coverage to a hospital in the developed world or close to your home. In addition we purchase AirMed, which can send a medical team via helicopter to stabilize your condition and evacuate you in the event of a severe injury or medical emergency situation. www.airmed.com If you take regular medication, carry an extra supply (or additional prescriptions) in case of emergency or delays when returning to your home country.

Sophisticated, high-ticket and high-tech Western medicine is not always necessary. **Bob:** I needed a quick fix for a broken tooth in Bali. Our guide took us to a lovely clinic in a home-temple compound, with gardens, open-air waiting room, and the traditional Balinese offerings of flowers and

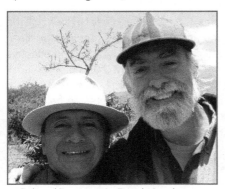

incense. He delivered quality dental care at a fraction of what I would have paid in the U.S.

In many areas of the world, you can find excellent alternative medical care while traveling: acupuncture in Asia (even in place of anesthesia for surgery), Ayurveda in India, homeopathy in India, and Heilpraktikers in Germany.

Bob and Don Joaquin, Ecuadorian shaman

Consider visiting a local, indigenous healer or shaman. Indigenous cultures have long traditions of healing, sometimes thousands of years old in places like India, China, Africa, South America, Australia, New Zealand, New Guinea, Polynesia and Siberia, and in most other parts of the developing world. *Curanderos* and shamans connect with and draw assistance and power from the local flora and fauna, the spirits of animals and ancestors, the energies of the earth, volcanoes, mountains, rivers, and lakes. They can journey to other planes of existence, or other parts of the planet to find what is needed for healing, or to understand the problems that the patient presents. These mysterious healers often chant and drum rhythmically, and may use hallucinogenic plants to access altered states of consciousness for healing.

In Bali we were taken to an elderly healer who diagnosed by poking a sharp stick in the side of each of the toes, looking for the reflex point corresponding to the ailing organ. When he touched a sensitive spot, the pain was startling, producing momentary levitation of the entire body. In Ecuador, we were sprayed, from the mouth of the shaman, with cane liquor

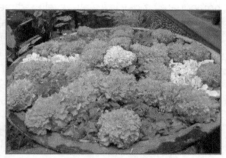

Balinese flower offerings

and various and sundry herbal waters. The chill of the alcohol bath was soon quelled by the warmth of the six-foot flame resulting from spraying the liquor through a candle. An experience to remember!

Bob: I have twice visited the internationally-renowned Brazilian medium and healer, John of God, who works with spirit doctors and saints, whom he channels to perform psychic surgery. Up to 500 patients a day visit, from all over the world, many with cancer and other serious illnesses. During my last pilgrimage there, I found myself sitting in the same room with Oprah and her film crew. There are probably mile-long lines now, thanks to the publicity!

Homeopathic Medicine

WHAT IS HOMEOPATHY?

Homeopathy is form of natural medicine developed over 200 years ago by Samuel Hahnemann, a practicing German physician, medical translator, and scientist. Hahnemann was steeped in the medical literature of his time, as well as ancient and current medical techniques. His mission was to find a simpler, less harmful form of treatment than the bloodletting, leeches and harsh medicinal treatments of the early 19th century. He succeeded, and homeopathy today is a well-developed medical science and art. It is used for both acute and chronic illness, and has remained consistently effective since Hahnemann's time. It is enjoyed by millions of people throughout the world, primarily in Europe, North America, South America and India.

Homeopathy gained its claim to fame in the European cholera and typhoid epidemics of the 1820s and 1830s and in the devastating flu pandemic in the U.S. of 1918. The results speak for themselves: a 30%-60% rate of mortality with conventional care compared to 1% with homeopathy! Homeopathy provided relief to American troops during World War I. By the turn of the 19th century, homeopathy enjoyed enjoyed significant popularity in the U.S.: over 20 homeopathic medical colleges, 100 hospitals, close to 1,000 homeopathic pharmacies, and one out of every five or six physicians was a homeopath. After 1910, homeopathy diminished in popularity in this country until its resurgence in the 1970s, however it continued to spread throughout the world. During the 35 years we have studied and practiced homeopathy, the skeptics have never been so vociferous as during the past year. The harmful influence has been felt particularly in the U.K., where Helios pharmacy, one of the best in the world, has been forced to call their homeopathic medicines "confectionaries." We hope that this wave of frivolous harassment passes, and that those who enjoy practicing and using homeopathy can continue to do so freely.

Homeopathic medicine can be a very effective treatment for first aid, acute, and chronic medical conditions. In this book we cover treatment for first aid and acute problems that could potentially affect you, or spoil your trip. By taking along a small, lightweight kit of homeopathic medicines, you will be very well equipped to treat most illnesses and injuries during your travels.

HOW HOMEOPATHY IS UNIQUE

Homeopathy is unique, even among other forms of natural medicine:

- The same substance that causes a set of symptoms in a healthy person can *cure* those same symptoms in someone who is ill.

- One single medicine treats the whole person constitutionally for chronic problems.

- Less is more: the more the medicine is diluted, the stronger it is.

- *Any* substance from nature can be made into a homeopathic medicine. There are over 3500 medicines, made from substances as diverse as table salt, gold, dolphin's milk, diamond, eagle, and hydrogen.

- Homeopathy treats people, not diseases.

- A medicine is chosen on the basis of the *totality* of symptoms (the

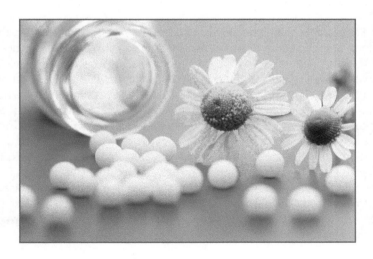

whole person). In the case of an acute illness, this includes whatever has *changed* since the person became acutely ill. So 5 different people with the same illness may need 5 different medicines.

- The prescription is based on what is *unique* (homeopaths say "strange, rare, and peculiar") about the symptoms.

- Homeopathy is safe even for newborns, pregnant women, the elderly, highly sensitive people, or those with compromised immune systems.

- A single dose of a homeopathic medicine, if given in a high potency, can last for months, or even longer.

- The medicines are very inexpensive when compared to prescription drugs.

WHAT ARE HOMEOPATHIC MEDICINES?

Homeopathic medicines are tiny, highly diluted, yet powerful doses of natural substances. They are very safe and effective when chosen correctly and given in the correct dosage. They are available in pellet form or as liquids. The majority of medicines come from the mineral and plant kingdoms, and the rest from the animal kingdom, but they can be made from literally anything in nature. Each of these substances has the ability to cause, and therefore treat, a unique set of physical, mental, and emotional symptoms.

For example, the homeopathic medicine, *Apis mellifica,* made from the honeybee, can be used to treat bee stings. It can also be used effectively to treat any condition that is similar to a bee sting, where there is inflammation, swelling redness and stinging pain. Conjunctivitis, an eye infection, often has similar symptoms, with swollen lids, red eyes and stinging pain. A few doses of *Apis* when your eyes start stinging, swelling and watering can often stop the conjunctivitis in its tracks. *Rhus toxicodendron*, derived from poison ivy, can be used in first aid to treat poison ivy, but is also a common medicine for sports injuries and arthritis. It is indicated when the joint pain is better from motion and stretching, and accompanied by inflammation and swelling, *Rhus tox.* will rapidly improve the situation. It is also a common medicine for herpes zoster or shingles, which has painful, itching spots along nerve roots, and symptoms that are quite similar to an exposure to poison ivy.

No two medicinal substances in homeopathy are exactly alike, in terms of the symptoms they treat, but substances that are similar to one another in nature also can have similarities medicinally. For chronic illness, we choose from among several thousand medicines, based on a complex, and highly organized system of classification. For first aid and acute conditions, it is usually possible to choose between a few medicines.

Homeopathic medicines are made and sold by homeopathic pharmacies. You can also find them at health food stores, pharmacies, online, or by consulting a homeopathic practitioner.

HOW TO CHOOSE AND GIVE A HOMEOPATHIC MEDICINE

1. Take the Case
You can take your own case or the case of someone else who is suffering. The object of taking the case is to identify symptoms, and to make a note of:

- What makes the symptoms feel better or worse

- What makes the sufferer feel better or worse

- Any other changes that have occurred since the injury or illness began

Think of this process as "Look, Listen, and Ask." The object is to develop a description of the illness that you can then compare to the descriptions in this book. Even though an illness has a name, such as influenza or migraine headache, homeopathy treats people, not symptoms.

Each person experiences symptoms uniquely, and it is in this uniqueness that the characteristic symptoms of the homeopathic medicine are found. No two people experience the same illness in exactly the same way, though there are common symptoms that most people may have with a certain condition, such as urinary pain with a bladder infection, or severe head pain with a migraine. You are trying to find what is unique to each particular problem.

2. Put Together the Acute Symptom Picture and Select a Medicine
After taking the case, think about what symptoms are the most unusual,

intense, and clear. Can you see any pattern in what you have heard and observed? Look at the description of the homeopathic medicines listed under the condition. Even if it is not a perfect match, choose the medicine that has symptoms closest to what you have seen and heard from the patient. **The BOLDED MEDICINES** indicated for each travel health problem are the ones most commonly used.

Look, Listen, and Ask

- Is the illness life threatening? If so, call 911 or other emergency care and administer first aid in the meantime. You can also put *Arnica* pellets under the tongue or give a few drops of Rescue Remedy.

- Ask what happened and get specific symptoms.

- What is the mental and emotional picture? (Is there a change in mental abilities or is there a feeling of anxiety, anger, fright, or grief?)

- Which symptoms are the most intense?

- Which symptoms are the most unusual?

- What symptoms can you actually observe?

- What makes the symptoms better or worse? (Motion, position, activity, noise, light, hot or cold, or any other factor?)

- Are the symptoms right-sided or left-sided?

- Any strong cravings for food or drink? (If so, hot or cold?)

- Any change in temperature? (Chills, fever, perspiration?)

- Any discharges? (Color, texture, smell, acrid or bland?)

3. Administer the Medicine

If you have selected a single medicine from the 5 or so medicines listed for your condition, take as follows:

Taking the Medicines

- Tap two globules or a few tiny pellets, into the cap, spoon, or onto a small piece of paper (3 to 5 tiny pellets is sufficient. More will not make you better faster and will waste the medicine, though refills are available.)

- Place the globules or pellets under your tongue or into your mouth. Let them dissolve.

- The recommended frequency to take a dose varies with the pace of the condition and the potency. With intense, rapid-paced illnesses such as fevers, ear infections, and bladder infections, you should see a marked response within half an hour after the first dose. With more slow-paced conditions like a dental abscess or a cold, take the well-matched medicine every 2-4 hours, until you see an improvement.

- If your symptoms seem to get worse at first, wait to take another dose until the aggravation goes away, then follow the instructions above.

- If your symptoms have changed for the better, only take another dose if the symptoms that have improved start to get worse again.

- If the symptoms change significantly or if the first medicine chosen did not significantly change your symptoms after 2 doses, see if another homeopathic medicine matches the same or new symptoms more exactly. If so take the new medicine as above.

THE SAVVY TRAVELER'S GUIDE TO HOMEOPATHY AND NATURAL MEDICINE

WHAT TO EXPECT FROM FIRST AID AND ACUTE HOMEOPATHY

You should notice improvement in your symptoms within 6-24 hours, and often much sooner. You may need to take doses of your medicine whenever your symptoms begin to relapse after improvement.

If your symptoms change, and the medicine you have been taking no longer seems to work, you may need to look for a different medicine that is a better match for the new symptom picture. If taking a combination medicine, if you see no results within a day, either try to find the single best medicine for your condition, or use other natural or conventional treatment.

Homeopathic medicine does not usually have side effects. But, if you take a homeopathic medicine that does not match your symptoms well over and over, even when there is no improvement, you could temporarily acquire symptoms of the medicine you are taking. This is called a *proving*. If it occurs, stop the medicine and the symptoms should go away, usually in less than 24 hours. As a last resort, you can antidote the homeopathic medicine by applying an aromatic compound containing camphor, such as BENGAY, Carmex or Blistex to your skin, but we have only needed to do that with patients a few times in 30+ years, so it is highly unlikely you will.

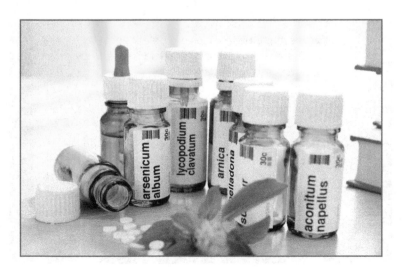

Homeopathic Practice Cases

If you are not familiar with treating yourself and others for first aid and acute conditions, the following cases will give you some practice. (See page 220 for correct answers.) You are most likely to have the 30C potency in your homeopathic kit. To know how often to repeat a medicine, see page 61. As experienced homeopathic practitioners, we carry kits with higher potencies, such as 200C and 1M, but the correct medicine will work in any potency. You may just need to repeat it more often.

1. Burn

A patient family was vacationing at a mountain cabin in Montana. Their five-year-old daughter, Molly, sat, without thinking, on top of a hot wood stove. She burned her bottom badly to an awesome shade of bright red, with big blisters. Her panicked parents called us on their cell phone to ask what to give from their homeopathic kit, with their child loudly bawling in the background. He replied immediately: "Give Molly_____30C from your kit. Within a half hour she had calmed down, the blisters had diminished in size, and the skin was less weepy and painful. By the next day, after several more doses, the child was clearly on the mend, and could even sit down. Molly completely recovered with no scarring. (See BURNS, page 81)

2. Food Poisoning

Bob: While in Mumbai, India we ordered *thali* plate dinners, a circle of small metal bowls with a variety of spicy veg or non-veg delicacies, and a dessert like rice pudding. I also ordered my favorite drink, a *mango lassi* (yogurt drink with fresh or canned mango). It tasted a bit "off." By that evening, I was crouched in front of the toilet, moaning, having profusely vomited 6 or 7 times. The nausea was extreme, with a strong urge to vomit, which I did over and over, until there was nothing left. Then came the dry heaves, until I took _____. Within 15 minutes the vomiting subsided, I fell asleep, and was fine the next morning. (See FOOD POISONING, page 124)

3. Insect Bite

Judyth: We were at a friend's cabin in northern Chile while editing this book. I woke with my right eyelid swollen from a likely spider bite. I immediately took a dose of _____ and I totally forgot about the swelling. It must have been gone within minutes. I wish I had known about this remedy when I was visiting Brazil in 1970. At that time I woke up with the whole right side of my face swollen like a balloon. I couldn't even open my eye. The family with whom I was staying immediately called their family doc, who came out and gave me an injection of some kind or other, which took care of it. (See INSECT BITES AND STINGS, page 161)

4. Bladder Infection

Angelica called us on a Saturday for help with acute pain due to a bladder infection. She was frantic because she needed to get on a plane for the East Coast in a few hours. She was a schoolteacher and had gotten so involved with her classroom the day before that she had forgotten to go to the bathroom as well as not having drunk any water all day. She complained of severe burning pain where the pee comes out (the urethra). It seemed worse just as she finished peeing. We advised her to take _____ from her kit, to drink lots of water, and, if convenient, to get cranberry capsules or drink diluted cranberry juice or concentrate. She emailed us that evening, having arrived much relieved in New York. The pain had gone away within 15 minutes after the first dose. She knew to take another dose if it returned, but it wasn't necessary. (See BLADDER INFECTION, page 77)

5. Acute Appendicitis

Bob: A few years out of naturopathic school, I developed a sudden, severe, sharp pain in my right abdomen, midway between my belly button and pelvic bones. I felt feverish and sweaty, and the pain was so intense that I could only lie in one position, curled up on my right side. Whenever I tried to move or change position, the pain was excruciating. I got up with great difficulty, hobbled over to my homeopathic kit and took _____ . Within 30 minutes the pain began to go away. When it returned later that night, I took another dose, which again gave relief. Over the next 24 hours I took three more doses, which worked each time.

I suspected appendicitis, but I didn't consult a doctor because the pain did not return until months later. This time the medicine worked only briefly. I was hospitalized with a burst appendix, had an appendectomy, and was given IV antibiotics for 5 days. I took the homeopathic medicine *Staphysagria* (Stavesacre) for the after-effects of abdominal surgery, and recovered fully over the next two weeks.

I admit that it would have been much wiser to consult a doctor after the first episode. I would have still needed the appendectomy, but could have been spared the high drama, especially since peritonitis from a ruptured appendix can prove fatal. (See STOMACH ACHES AND ACUTE ABDOMINAL PAIN, page 205)

6. Traveler's Diarrhea
Judyth: While sitting in a homeopathic classroom in Mumbai, India, I felt a sudden rumbling vibration in my abdomen. I ran out the door in desperate search of a bathroom. The pain was intense, with tremendous pressure, as if my gut would burst at any moment. The diarrhea shot out, into the toilet, like water from a fire hose. I raced to our hotel room and immediately took _____. Within minutes, my noisy abdomen quieted and the diarrhea did not recur. (See DIARRHEA, page 105)

7. Cold
On a pilgrimage to Konya, Turkey, our group leader leader came down with what she referred to as "a stinking cold." She sneezed incessantly, and her nose was perpetually dripping with clear, thin, watery mucus, requiring countless tissues. She was thoroughly miserable. We gave her a dose of _____. It worked very quickly and she was impressed at how much better she felt the next day. Unfortunately, a number of other members came down with an even worse version of cold and cough. We were busy choosing medicines from our kits for the next week. (See COLDS, page 88)

8. Ear Infections and Teething
A young mother who was a patient of ours called us in tears from her in-laws' in Ohio. "We are visiting my husband's parents and our seven-month-old toddler, Sammy, just came down with a raging ear infection. He's cutting his first tooth and he is like a different child. Normally sweet and good-natured, he is terribly fussy, has a 100F (37.8C) fever, and he is inconsolable with pain.

He keeps pulling on his right ear. We've never seen him like this. Whatever we offer him, he seems to want something else. My mother-in-law is pushing us to call a pediatrician, who I know will want to give him antibiotics. Help!" We instructed her to give Sammy _____ from her kit, and assured her that he would feel better within a few minutes to a couple of hours maximum. She emailed us later that day to thank us. "Sammy is so much better. He went right to sleep after the dose. When he woke up, three hours later, he was in much better spirits and his ear seemed fine." We told the mom to give him a repetition of the dose if he relapsed. (See EAR INFECTIONS, page 111)

9. Airplane Anxiety

Monica hated flying. It made her feel completely out of control. "My heart starts to beat wildly, my forehead and palms sweat, and I feel sure that the plane will crash and I will die. I am a sales rep and need to fly once a month. It is the worst time for me. I start dreading it a week in advance. I'm afraid I will have to change careers if I can't get a handle on my anxiety!" We told Monica to take_____ the morning of the flight and, again, during the flight if needed. She reported that she felt far better before boarding the plane, but took another dose prior to takeoff "just in case." She felt 90% better, and will surely follow these recommendations again whenever she flies. (See: FEAR OF FLYING, page 117)

10. Hay Fever

Antonio was miserable every time he visited Sacramento, California, where his parents lived. He had invested in every over-the-counter antihistamine he could find, but none brought long-lasting relief. "My nose runs constantly and the itching and tingling in my nose and upper palate drives me crazy. My eyes are red and they burn. But the absolute worst is the constant, violent sneezing. It helps temporarily to go inside, but the minute I go back out, it starts all over again. When I help my dad by taking over the lawn mowing, I feel like I'm going to die." Antonio needed _____ . He takes one dose each time he visits his parents, and is a happy camper, or should we say, happy mower. (See: HAY FEVER, page 140)

Travel Health Problems

Our goal is that this book be small and light enough to easily slip into a suitcase, backpack, or daypack, or access the e-book on your phone or tablet, so the intros are short and sweet. You can look up more detailed info online if needed. We do, where appropriate, give first aid or emergency guidelines. We have included most of the conditions that appear in our larger-format *Homeopathic Self-Care: The Quick and Easy Guide for the Whole Family*, with a much more abbreviated text. You will find all of the first aid conditions that you are most likely to encounter, most common acute illnesses, and a handful of the most important and common tropical infectious diseases. There is far too much to cover regarding rare conditions limited to isolated parts of the world. We have three decades of experience as natural doctors, but nearly none in tropical medicine. We leave that to the experts. You will find homeopathic treatment for many tropical diseases in *The Natural Medicine Guide for Travel and Home* by Richard Pitt (see Bibliography).

We have included anecdotes from our own travels and experience in hopes of making the book more friendly and personal.

HOMEOPATHY

We include simple, easy-to-use indications for which homeopathic medicine to choose. **THE BOLDED MEDICINES** are the most commonly used ones for each conditions, though you want to find the medicine that best fits your particular symptoms. It is easy to travel with a small, lightweight homeopathic kit. We have included ALL of the medicines, or remedies, that we feel are indispensable for each condition, whether or not you are likely to find them easily. Often the one that you need will be included in our companion Homeopathic Self-Care Medicine Kit or another travel kit. In other cases, you can either order them from a homeopathic pharmacy in advance, just in case, or, if you happen to be traveling in a country that sells them (India, the U.S., U.K., much of Europe, and some other parts of the world) you can wait and buy as needed.

The key to homeopathic prescribing is to **HAVE THE MEDICINES YOU NEED** at your fingertips. **DON'T LEAVE HOME WITHOUT THEM**. Read the sections in our book that explain how to decide what you need, how to administer, and when to change medicines. That way, being familiar with how to use homeopathy, you can act quickly when needed.

 PREVENTION

These tips will hopefully keep you free of the problem altogether.

 MORE NATURAL TIPS

These are easy naturopathic recommendations to use either in addition to the homeopathic medicines, or on their own. Most of what we mention in this section is readily available or can be taken along with you on your trip. We carry six months worth of nutritional supplements with us to Chile in Zip-lock bags. Just be sure to put the preservative plugs in the bag as well. If you are in indigenous areas, the locals can surely suggest local herbs and other remedies that are tried and true and work quickly.

 LIFESAVERS

Just as the name suggests, these are invaluable tips in potentially life-and-death situations.

 TRIPSAVERS

Many a trip is canceled or spoiled unnecessarily when just a simple piece of advice could have saved the day. These suggestions often work more quickly and effectively than conventional medicine.

ALLERGIC REACTIONS

Mild allergic reactions (swelling, redness, itching and inflammation) are a bother, but severe reactions can provoke anaphylaxis (significant itching and swelling of the lymph nodes, nose and ears, with respiratory arrest), and can lead to rapid death. Hay fever is a reaction to pollens from grasses, trees, or flowers. Symptoms include a watery nasal discharge, sneezing, itchy nose, eyes, and mouth, headache, and irritability.

HOMEOPATHY

- **Apis** (Honeybee): Swelling. Redness, stinging pains. Better from cold packs. Useful first aid for bee stings.

- **Allium cepa** (Onion): Symptoms just like when you peel an onion: nose runs like a faucet and eyes stream.

- *Carbolic acid:* Anaphylaxis, especially after bee stings. Shock from allergic reaction.

- **Euphrasia** (Eyebright): Symptoms focus on eyes. Watery eyes, nose.

- *Rhus tox.* Short for *Rhus toxicodendron* (Poison ivy): Blistery eruptions with itching and joint pain or stiffness.

- **Sabadilla** (Mexican grass): Violent sneezing in fits.

- *Urtica urens* (Stinging nettle): Nettle-like stinging. Reaction to shellfish.

Judyth: I was out in the garden picking raspberries and got stung by the surrounding nettles. I took a dose of *Urtica urens* and the stinging was relieved almost immediately. It happened to be the same night that we had our first healing session with an Ecuadorian shaman, a part of which was being flogged by fresh nettles. Poor Bob was up till 3AM, too uncomfortable to sleep. I felt fine after ten minutes, thanks to having taken the *Urtica* earlier that day!

PREVENTION

- Wraparound sunglasses can be useful to stop pollen from entering your eyes when you are outdoors.

- Shower, change clothes, and dry clothing indoors to reduce contact with pollen.

MORE NATURAL TIPS

- Soaking in a bathtub of warm water with a cup of baking soda or finely- ground oatmeal can reduce itching of the skin considerably.

- Buffered Vitamin C 500mg every two hours, up to 3000mg/day, or apple cider vinegar, mixed with water, can reduce acidity and take the edge off the allergic symptoms.

- We use with patients natural antihistamines such as quercetin (a bioflavonoid from the oak tree) capsules or nasal spray, and *Euphrasia* (eyebright) eye drops, if a local natural pharmacy is available.

- On occasion, when other homeopathic medicines have not worked, we have used the homeopathic medicine, *Histaminum*.

 LIFESAVERS

- If you know that you have severe allergic reactions, use an Epi Pen (epinephrine) or SEEK EMERGENCY CARE IMMEDIATELY! For swelling try *Apis*. If you have any tendency to anaphylactic shock, we suggest that you carry both *Apis* and *Carbolic acid*, since the latter is hard to find.

- **Judyth:** We had just arrived at a beautiful ashram in Southern India, and I was lying in the grass relaxing. Suddenly my nose, throat, and lymph nodes began to itch and swell, and I noticed a number of insect bites. We knew no one there, and I was reluctant to wait until the following morning to get help. I took *Apis* and went directly to the health center, where I was given an epinephrine shot. Better safe than sorry in rural India! I was fine within a few minutes.

- If highly prone to severe reactions, wear a bracelet or tag to alert others in case of emergency.

 TRIPSAVERS

- If allergy-prone, research your destination to avoid going at the height of the pollen season. Even a week or two can make all the difference.

ALTITUDE SICKNESS (Acute Mountain Sickness, or AMS)

The name of the game is "acclimatize". Arriving a couple of days early to your high-altitude destination can make all the difference in the world between a great experience and a miserable one. It takes about three weeks to fully acclimatize. The higher you go, the thinner the air, the less available oxygen, and the more terrible you are likely to feel. The risk of AMS generally begins a little over an altitude of 8,000 feet (2,500 meters). Anyone of any age and health status may suffer. Hiking above 3,500 feet (1100 meters) affects about half of all trekkers, 5% seriously, especially if you remain at that altitude for more than six hours.

Mild symptoms include headache, shortness of breath, loss of appetite, nausea and vomiting, fatigue, irritability, and difficulty sleeping. If symptoms are severe, you may experience breathlessness, even at rest, coughing up pink, frothy sputum, severe headache, double vision, sleepiness, and unsteadiness. Severe AMS can be LIFE THREATENING and requires IMMEDIATE emergency medical attention.

HOMEOPATHY

Homeopathy is quite effective in preventing and treating altitude sickness. We recently traveled to the Atacama Desert in the Chilean Andes and were able to walk around comfortably, though briefly (with down jackets and mufflers) at 5,265 meters (17,274 feet), fully enjoying the view of eleven volcanoes! One of our patients used it very successfully during her ascent of Mt. Rainier. *Coca* is available only in certain countries from homeopathic pharmacies.

- *Arsenicum album* (Arsenic): If you don't have *Coca*. Anxiety, restlessness, heart palpitations, chilliness, weakness from slight exertion, and fear of death.

- **Coca** (Erythroxylon coca): "The mountaineer's medicine." Specific for altitude sickness. Symptoms are difficulty breathing, heart palpitations, anxiety, and insomnia. We take it on the plane when we fly to a very high destination, as well as the morning that we start to climb. We use a 200C or 1M potency of this medicine, but 30C will likely be fine for you.

PREVENTION

- Be in the best possible physical condition before trekking.

- Allow a couple of days to acclimatize and rest after arriving at a high altitude.

- Ascend slowly and gradually. Spend two to three nights at each elevation gain of 3000 feet (about 1000 meters) while trekking.

- Climb high and sleep low. Sleep at lower altitudes than you climb each day.

- Do not climb solo.

- Drink lots of fluids to prevent dehydration and avoid alcohol.

- If you develop symptoms, wait until they subside before ascending any further.

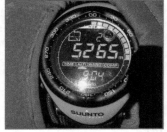

Our guide's altimeter in the Atacama Desert, Chile

MORE NATURAL TIPS

- *Coca* tea (mate de coca) is widely available around Machu Picchu and other high areas in South America, and helps acclimatization. The indigenous Peruvians may appear to be suffering from the mumps, but they are actually chewing wads of coca leaves to keep up their energy.

LIFESAVERS

- Descend immediately if your symptoms are severe, persist, or worsen.

- Do NOT be too macho or embarrassed to admit that you are having symptoms of AMS or hesitate to tell your trekking companions.

- Do not hesitate to use oxygen if you are having trouble breathing.

- Do NOT drive a vehicle if you are dizzy, drowsy, disoriented, or ill.

TRIPSAVERS

- If you follow the guidelines of safe ascent, medication should not be necessary. Acetazolamide (Diamox) is a conventional medication, which can be used to prevent or treat mild AMS, but it won't help with severe AMS, and it does have side effects.

ANIMAL BITES AND SCRATCHES

Bites are a big concern in many areas of the world. Street dogs are common in Latin America, Asia and elsewhere. In rural areas, dogs are rarely contained, vaccinated, or spayed/neutered, and may be trained to protect farm animals and guard dwellings against intruders, even with their lives. Dogs and cats may not be considered pets and, even worse, may be part of the local cuisine. Rodents are rampant in many areas, both rural and urban, and bats may be prevalent as well. Risks include not only rabies, but also secondary bacterial infection, which can be quite serious. If your flesh is broken, unless you can be sure the animal is free of rabies, you must assume it is not and proceed with shots.

FIRST apply strong alcohol or topical iodine preparation to kill the potential rabies virus, do NOT close the wound with stitches. Seek medical care as soon as possible. If you are out in the sticks, you do have a window of at least a week, but since rabies can be fatal, the sooner you seek out anti-rabies injections, the better.

Symptoms of rabies infection include fever, headache, nausea, and sore throat, followed by pain and burning around the bite, anxiety, extreme sensitivity to light and sound. There is the classic hydrophobia (fear of water resulting from painful throat spasms upon drinking), and foaming at the mouth, followed, finally, by convulsions and coma resulting in death.

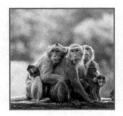

Besides canines, you may find yourself bitten by a monkey, or other mammal, or by a sea animal, such as a jellyfish, stingray, or eel. While relaxing on a beach near *Yelapa*, Mexico, a child let out a scream, after being bitten by an eel. Local fishermen had boned their catch on the beach, the eel came to scarf up the leftovers, and the innocent child got in its way. The mom, a pediatrician, was frantic. Fortunately a savvy local knew to apply lemon juice to the area, the pain subsided quickly, and the child was fine within ten minutes.

HOMEOPATHY

- *Apis* (Honeybee): Swelling around the bite is the main symptom. Also redness and stinging pains. Better from cold packs.

- **Ledum** (Marsh tea): Animal bites, especially deep puncture wounds. Area around the bite is cold to the touch and feels better from immersing in ice-cold water. Burning pain may also be present.

- *Lyssin* (Rabies, Hydrophobinum): Suspicion of rabies infection.

- **Medusa** (Jellyfish) is the best choice for a jellyfish sting and can be ordered ahead from a homeopathic pharmacy. *Ledum* is 2nd.

PREVENTION

- The rabies vaccine needs refrigeration, so it is difficult to take with you.

- Sleep under a mosquito net in rural, bat-inhabited areas, making sure to cover your feet, since they tend to bite in between the toes.

- If you plan to travel or spend extended time in remote, rural areas, check first to find out the rabies status of the region.

- If you are traveling with your dog: Many countries require rabies vaccines at least 30 days and no more than one year before travel. This is the case even though the veterinary conventional wisdom indicates that rabies vaccines are needed every three years at most, perhaps only once in the animal's life. Some countries, including the U.S., are beginning to allow rabies titers as sufficient evidence that further vaccination in unnecessary.

- Stay out of waters inhabited seasonally by box jellyfish, such as the Great Barrier Reef of Australia. These mollusks can be deadly.

MORE NATURAL TIPS

- *Calendula, Calendula-Hypericum*, and colloidal silver can all be used topically on bites to reduce the risk of infection and sepsis.

- For jellyfish stings: Get out of the water. If in non-tropical areas, wash the area with seawater to deactivate stinging cells. In tropical waters, rinse immediately with vinegar or lemon juice rather than fresh or tap water, which can reactivate stinging cells, for at least 30 seconds. Or, if vinegar is unavailable, use a solution of baking soda. Soak the area in hot water for at least 20 minutes or, if not possible, use cold packs.

LIFESAVERS

- A suspected or known rabies bite requires anti-rabies injections, regardless of the cost. In addition, you will need a rabies immunoglobulin injection if you were not previously vaccinated, which may be expensive. Imported human vaccines are far preferable to locally made ones, especially in rural areas, due to possible infection risks. This will likely mean an immediate trip to the nearest major city. Rabies infection IS TREATABLE before the above symptoms appear, which can be days, months, or even longer. Once the severe symptoms listed above appear, it is FATAL. GET HELP quickly if bitten, except in the case of a domesticated dog, that you can be sure was vaccinated.

- Anti-venom is administered for box jellyfish stings. Hospitalization may be required. This is a *life-threatening* emergency!

TRIPSAVERS

- If immediate medical help is not available, seek out a course of treatment with antibiotics, generally with penicillin or erythromycin in the meantime, until you can obtain the anti-rabies injections. While taking antibiotics, eat fermented foods or take an antibiotic-resistant probiotic (such as *Saccharomyces boulardii*) to protect your gut flora.

BED BUGS

These insects were around during the time of the ancient Greeks and Romans, and there has been a resurgence of them in the U.S. in recent years. If you are a budget traveler, or perhaps any traveler, you may run into this unpleasant problem. These small, reddish-brown, flat, oval, parasitic insects live in mattresses and cracks in walls and feed on blood. The bites, which do itch, show up in a line of two or three on the face, arms, ankles, butt, or anywhere that flesh is exposed. They are mainly active at night and go unnoticed except for the bites. They have a characteristic smell like rotten raspberries.

HOMEOPATHY

- *Cimex* (Bed bug): There is very little information about this medicine, but being the source material, it could be helpful. Not easy to obtain except from a well stocked homeopathic pharmacy.

- *Ledum* (Marsh tea): Insect bites in general. Area can be cold to the touch and feel better from ice or cold applications.

- *Sulphur* (Sulfur): The best bet, and it will be in any kit. Nagging itching worse warmth, heat of the bed, and bathing.

PREVENTION

- Avoid sleeping in dirty bedrooms.

- Use sleeping bags or sleeping sacks. We stayed at a dive of a hotel one night in Calcutta before getting up at 5AM the next morning to see Mother Theresa at mass. The hotel was SO filthy (with people lying out in the hallway sleeping as well) that we were afraid to get under the sheets. We slept on top of the bed on our sleeping bags!

- Conventional wisdom is to spray furniture and wall cracks with insecticide but this "cure" may be worse than the original problem and leads to super bugs that eventually are resistant to all efforts to kill them.

- A mosquito net impregnated with permethrin may help.

MORE NATURAL TIPS

- Bed Defense is an aromatic herbal product with favorable reviews. www.beddefense.com

BLADDER INFECTIONS (Cystitis)

Bladder infections may not be fatal, but, along with kidney stones, appendicitis, and toothaches, they can be near the top of the pain scale. Waiting too long without urinating is a common predisposing factor. So is not drinking enough water, so make sure you have a water bottle within reach and keep reminding yourself to drink. Frequent bathroom trips are far better than suffering a UTI. Urgency and frequency are the first indicators, followed by pain.

HOMEOPATHY

- *Apis* (Honeybee): Stinging, burning pain. Scalding urine. Swelling of urethra.

- *Berberis*: Pains, stitches or bubbling. Copious urine and frequent urging.

- **Cantharis** (Spanish fly): Extreme pain. Rapid onset. Bloody urine (sometimes). Tremendous urging, frequency, and restlessness. Frenzied with the pain. Burning sensations before, during and after urinating.

- **Sarsaparilla** (Wild licorice): Severe pain in the urethra at the close of urination. Very commonly needed for women with UTIs.

- **Staphysagria** (Stavesacre): Burning in the urethra on urinating. Onset of UTI after overdoing sex, or after sex with a new partner. Watch out you mile-high clubbers—airplanes are dehydration machines!

PREVENTION

- Drink as much water as possible.

- Urinate promptly when you have the urge.
- If you are a woman, and know you will be trekking or traveling in areas where you can't bare your bottom to pee, wear long skirts and relieve yourself wherever you can.
- Know at least one word in the local language: bathroom!
- If prone, take cranberry capsules preventively.
- If certain foods or drinks increase your risk, avoid them.
- Be even more proactive about all of the above after more frequent sex than usual.
- If you tend to UTIs, take with you your treatment of choice preventively.

MORE NATURAL TIPS

- Herbal formulas containing Oregon grape, bearberry, corn silk, and bucchu can be quite helpful. Tinctures have the quickest action.
- If you can't find cranberry juice, citrus juice may relieve symptoms.
- In a pinch, try 1 teaspoon of bicarbonate of soda in a glass of water.

LIFESAVERS

- Kidney infection can be very serious. You may be tempted to ignore UTI symptoms while traveling. Don't! Better to deal with a UTI early than be stuck in a dingy, dirty hospital in the middle of nowhere getting antibiotics. Back pain and a high fever are warning signs.

TRIPSAVERS

- Homeopathy can work amazingly quickly for UTIs. Regardless of which type of treatment you prefer, the sooner you get help, the better. It can make all the difference between a minor annoyance and a trip wrecker!
- If you have no access to a natural alternative, or have waited too long, as a last resort see a local physician and get a prescription for

antibiotics. Take either an antibiotic-resistant probiotic during the course of antibiotics (*Saccharomyces boulardii*), or take a probiotic or yogurt, after finishing the antibiotics, to replenish your gut flora.

BLEEDING

To stop bleeding, apply a constant, firm pressure to the wound for at least five minutes. A strip or butterfly band-aid is generally fine for superficial cuts. For more serious bleeding, place a clean gauze pad or cloth on the wound and apply even pressure, then check regularly to make sure bleeding has not recurred. Lie down. If it is a wound to the extremity, raise the limb above the heart to reduce the amount of blood loss. Death can result in minutes if the flow of blood is not arrested.

Judyth: I will never forget the poor Indian mother, lying helplessly on the street in Old Delhi, with a post-partum hemorrhage. She desperately needed I.V. fluid and hospitalization, but I was unable to summon emergency medical assistance. To my horror and helplessness, she died within half an hour.

HOMEOPATHY

- **Arnica** (Leopard's bane): Bleeding from trauma of any kind or from bruising. Refuses help.

- **Belladonna** (Deadly nightshade): Sudden, bright-red bleeding. Flushed face.

- **China** (Peruvian bark): Profuse bleeding leading to weakness and collapse. Pale face.

- *Crotalus horridus* (Rattlesnake): Bleeding from all openings of the body. Dark, un-clotted blood. Slow, oozing hemorrhages.

- *Ferrum metallicum* (Iron): Bright red hemorrhages with small clots. Bright red cheeks or pale face. Anemia after bleeding.

- *Phosphorus*: Fluid, non-clotted blood. Tendency to bleed easily. Small wounds bleed a lot.

PREVENTION

- If you have a known blood disorder, know your blood type and consider joining a trusted donor group abroad. If you plan to spend extended time in Africa, or other areas at high risk for AIDS, and will be doing rural health care, consider purchasing a personal-protection CPR/spill kit, which will help protect you from blood-borne pathogens if you have to do CPR on a patient who could have AIDS or other blood-borne illnesses.

MORE NATURAL TIPS

- A number of herbs, including common kitchen spices, can be helpful. Cinnamon, cayenne, and, if available, goldenseal, can be applied topically as a powder directly to the wound. Yarrow and shepherd's purse can be taken in tea or tincture form for hemorrhages.

LIFESAVERS

- Wear gloves when in contact with someone else's blood, especially when traveling in areas where AIDS is prevalent.

- If, due to trauma, surgery, or childbirth, you need a blood transfusion while traveling, make sure it is free from infection. Only accept blood that has been HIV-tested immediately before you receive it. Use IV fluid until you can be sure that the donor blood is safe.

- Sharks, bears, and other animals are attracted by blood. If you find yourself in such a dire circumstance, use the necessary precautions to minimize or stop the blood flow.

✈ TRIPSAVERS

- If you know that you tend to bleed heavily, check for anemia before your departure.

BURNS AND SUNBURN

First-degree: Redness, heat, swelling, and pain. Second-degree: All of the above, plus blistering and oozing. Third-degree: No blisters. Instead they appear charred black or waxy white and, possibly, numbness. Burns can be serious, even fatal, depending on the degree and the extent of the body area affected. Sun damage is cumulative. Early signs are sunburn, tan, and increased freckles and, later, wrinkling, sagging, and premature aging.

First Aid

Immerse the burned area in cold water. Cleanse gently with soap and water and/or an antiseptic in diluted tincture, cream or ointment form. *Calendula* is very effective. If not available, use an over-the-counter product.

- First-degree burns (redness only) can be left uncovered.

- Second-degree burns: Do *not* pop blisters, because they are protective.

- Cover with a non-adhesive dressing and wrap with gauze to keep in place. Change the dressing once every couple of days.

- Third-degree burns: These serious burns involve all layers of the skin and cause permanent tissue damage, involving even fat, muscle, and bone. Seek emergency care! In the meantime: Do NOT remove burned clothing, but do make sure the person is no longer in contact with or exposed to the fire, smoke, or heat. Do NOT immerse large, severe burns in cold water because it could result in hypothermia or shock. If there is no breathing, start CPR. Elevate the burned body part above the head. Cover the burned area with a clean moist cloth or sterile bandage.

- Burns are susceptible to tetanus.

HOMEOPATHY

- *Cantharis* (Spanish fly): Any burn, especially if intensely painful.

  Judyth: I scalded my hand badly with hot soup while ladling it into a container at our local food coop. A customer, who happened to be next to me and saw what happened, commented, "That looks really bad. You should get some help." I ran out to the car and took a dose of *Cantharis* 30C from our kit. The response was immediate. Upon checking out, I happened to run into the same woman, who inquired about my hand. I assured her, "It's all better now thanks to homeopathy."

- *Causticum* (Potassium hydrate): Deep burns. Slow-healing burns. Chemical or electrical burns. Burn wounds that reopen.
- *Phosphorus*: Electrical burns.
- *Urtica urens* (Stinging nettle): Scalds. First- or second-degree burns with nettle-like stinging, intense burning pains, and itching.

PREVENTION

- Pay attention, and be vigilant of children, around campfires, wood-stoves, and stoves.

MORE NATURAL TIPS

- Apply *Calendula* (marigold) tincture, diluted one part *Calendula* to three parts water topically for first- and second-degree burns. Or use Calendula cream or salve.
- *Aloe vera* juice, either directly from a leaf of the plant, or as a commercial preparation, is very helpful for burns.
- Honey is an ancient burn treatment (antiseptic and antibiotic properties). Slather on immediately. Pursue other treatment as needed.

LIFESAVERS

- Overexposure to sun over time can predispose to melanoma. Strong, irregular sun exposure is a greater risk factor than long-term exposure.
- Get immediate medical attention for third-degree burns or serious electrical burns.

TRIPSAVERS

- As the billboards blast, all over Australian beaches: Slip, slop, slap.

Slip on a shirt, slop on sunscreen, and slap on a hat. We would add a special sun block for the lips. Sunscreen is a highly controversial topic these days—look for a more in-depth discussion in our Sunscreen section (See page 47).

CANKER SORES

These are the small, sometimes extremely painful, sores on the inside of the mouth or tongue. They usually resolve on their own in a week or two, but are annoying and can put a damper on your gustatory enjoyment.

HOMEOPATHY

- **Borax**: Specific for hot, sensitive canker sores that bleed when touched. Worse from acidic, salty, spicy food. Canker sores in kids with thrush.

- *Mercurius* (Mercury): Inflammation and ulceration of the mouth with excess saliva, bad breath, and a metallic taste in the mouth. Worse from both hot and cold food or drinks. Spongy, bleeding gums and indentations around the side of the tongue.

- *Natrum muriaticum* (Sodium chloride): Canker sores inside the mouth. Cold sores on the lips. Sores burn when food touches them. Dry lips with a crack in the middle of the tongue. Desire for salt.

PREVENTION

- Avoid foods high in acid, such as tomatoes, citrus, and vinegar, if you are prone to canker sores.

MORE NATURAL TIPS

- Apply pharmaceutical-grade alum powder with a cotton swab several times a day.

CHICKEN POX

This acute viral disease, common in young children, is related to shingles. Though it is generally mild, it is very contagious, which can be a concern while traveling, and may cause scarring. Infrequent complications include shingles and secondary bacterial infections (usually *Staph* or *Strep*).

HOMEOPATHY

- *Antimonium crudum* (Antimony): Eruptions have a honey-like discharge or thick, hard, honey-colored scabs. Sores burn and itch. Worse in bed.

- *Croton tiglium* (Croton seed oil): Blister-like eruptions with violent, intense, painful itching. Scratching is painful.

- *Pulsatilla* (Windflower): Itchy sores that blister and crust. Whiny, clingy, weeping child who is not thirsty.

- **Rhus tox** (Poison ivy): The first remedy to consider. Intense itching causes restlessness.

PREVENTION

- As naturopathic physicians, we believe that it is healthier for a child to experience chicken pox than to be vaccinated against it.

- To prevent infection, keep sores clean and avoid scratching.

MORE NATURAL TIPS

- Let the rash emerge fully before treating it topically.

- An oatmeal bath or cream can reduce itching.

- Apply *Calendula* tincture diluted 3:1 with water to infected sores, then cover with clean bandage or gauze.

- A *Grindelia* and *Sarsaparilla* herbal spray can reduce itching.

- Boost the child's immune system with olive leaf, elderberry, echinacea, Vitamin C, zinc, Vitamin D.

- Limit sugar, dairy, and processed foods.

C

LIFESAVERS

- Do NOT give aspirin to a child with chicken pox because they may develop Reye's Syndrome, a potentially life-threatening brain and liver disease causing nausea, vomiting, mental dullness, memory loss, disorientation, and coma.

TRIPSAVERS

- If you can't find oatmeal or Calamine lotion, add 2 ounces baking soda to the bath water.

CHOLERA

There are 3 to 5 million cases of cholera a year, in 58 countries, resulting in over 100,000 deaths. Although about 80% of cases can be treated successfully through rehydration, it can be fatal within hours, in both adults and children. About 75% of those infected are asymptomatic. In severe cases, there is watery, gushing diarrhea, with "rice water" stools (white mucus flecks). Homeopathy became famous in the 1854 cholera epidemic, and is often effective.

HOMEOPATHY

- *Arsenicum album* (Arsenic): Intense vomiting and purging, body cold and burning. Diarrhea worse from eating or drinking. Restless, anxious.

- *Camphora* (Camphor): Intense weakness with icy cold, bluish face even before the vomiting and diarrhea. Coldness and collapse. Even the tongue is cold.

- *Carbo vegetabilis* (Vegetable charcoal): Too weak to move, lifeless. Cold. Wants to be fanned.

- **Cuprum** (Copper): Intense abdominal spasms and cramps, even in the extremities. Dry mouth, cold body, twitching. Vomiting without cold sweat.

- **Veratrum album** (White hellebore): Profuse, explosive, watery stools. Cold sweats and weakness after bowel movements. Inner burning but skin is cold.

PREVENTION

- Your likelihood of contracting cholera is very low provided that you take basic precautions with food and water. Seafood, including crustaceans and shellfish, infected by sewage, are a common source, and are best avoided unless they come from a clean source.

- Shellfish should be thoroughly cooked.

- Basic hygiene can prevent most infections. Cholera is known to affect the poorest of the poor, where clean water and sanitation is unavailable. Be especially careful in areas where the water system has been contaminated due to hurricanes, flooding, and other natural disasters.

MORE NATURAL TIPS

- Live yogurt, if tolerated, does wonders to replenish the intestinal flora.

- Ayurvedic medicine recommends lime or lemon juice daily, coconut water, onion, bitter melon juice, and holy basil in boiled water. Also recommended is rice water. Sounds homeopathic given the stools!

- If you acquire cholera in a developing country, use the indigenous treatment in addition to rehydrating.

- Use antibiotics if necessary.

LIFESAVERS

- If you begin to have gushing, watery diarrhea, increase your intake of fluids immediately. If it persists for more than a few hours and you feel weak, get help. We heard of a traveler who went to bed and died within two days. DO NOT take these symptoms lightly!

TRIPSAVERS

Judyth: I love *ceviche* (raw, marinated fish or shellfish). When I order it In Peru or Chile, I stick to clean restaurants rather than street stands.

COLD SORES (Herpes)

C

Crops of eruptions in the form of blisters, typically on or around the lips, caused by the Herpes Simplex virus. Numbness, tingling, and fatigue may precede the outbreak. The blisters may be swollen, and painful. They usually disappear on their own in one to two weeks, but can be uncomfortable and embarrassing.

HOMEOPATHY

- *Arsenicum album* (Arsenic): Cold sores with intense, burning pain of the lips. Worse from sour or acid fruit. Thirsty for frequent sips of cold water. Restless, anxious, despairing.

- *Hepar sulphuris* (Calcium sulfate): Exquisitely painful cold sores, especially to the touch and to the cold air. Generally irritable and extremely chilly.

- **Natrum muriaticum** (Sodium chloride): Cold sores on or near the lips. Lips are dry with a crack in the middle of the lower lip. After grief or hurt feelings or over-exposure to sun.

- **Rhus tox.** (Poison ivy): Several small, intensely itchy blisters. Burning. Filled with watery, yellowish fluid.

- *Sepia* (Cuttlefish): Eruptions around lips, corners of the mouth and inside the nose. Sufferer often has dark circles under their eyes. After hormonal changes (pregnancy, menses, menopause).

PREVENTION

- Avoid sharing utensils, drinking cups, towels, or other personal items used by a person with a cold sore.

- Avoid kissing or coming into contact with infected body fluids.

- Apply lip sunscreen to your lips to prevent sun-induced recurrences.

- Take Lysine 500mg/day preventively.

- Do not squeeze, pinch, or pick a cold sore. Wash your hands often after touching the eruption and do not touch your genitals or eyes.

- Eat foods that are higher in Lysine than Arginine: fish, chicken, beef, lamb, milk, cheese, beans, brewer's yeast, mung bean sprouts, and most fruits and vegetables. Avoid high Arginine foods, such as chocolate, carob, coconut, oats, whole wheat and white flour, peanuts, soybeans, and wheat germ.

- Toothbrushes can harbor the herpes virus. Buy a new toothbrush after the blister has formed and again after it has cleared up.

MORE NATURAL TIPS

- Apply a lemon balm lip pomade or ointment.

- Vitamin C 1000mg, Vitamin A 25,000 IU, and zinc 30mg/day.

- Take Lysine 500mg three times a day during an outbreak.

- Products containing real licorice may stop the virus (look for "licorice mass" in the ingredients). Or try a licorice powder paste.

TRIPSAVERS

- If you are traveling in a high-profile situation, where a visible herpes outbreak would be would be very embarrassing or poorly-timed, start taking Lysine 500mgthree times a day and avoid eating the Arginine-rich foods above.

COLDS (Upper Respiratory Infection)

Colds are minor, acute illnesses, but they are also one of the most common reasons for downtime while traveling. Resist the temptation to "let it run its course!" There are many things you can do for prevention and natural care to avoid getting sick, even if everyone around you is honking and hawking.

HOMEOPATHY

- *Aconite* (Monkshood): Colds that come on quickly, with a high fever, especially after exposure to cold, dry winds. Use during the first 24 hours. Restlessness.

- **Allium cepa** (Onion): Nose runs like a faucet. Drippy eyes, just like when you peel an onion. Sneezing. Nasal discharge burns but eye discharge is bland.

- *Arsenicum album* (Arsenic): Thin, burning discharge from nose, Very chilly. Anxious, nervous, restless. Worse when alone. Thirsty for sips of cold water.

- *Belladonna* (Deadly nightshade): Cold with high fever that comes on suddenly. Bright-red face, sore throat, throbbing headache. Worse right side.

- **Kali bichromicum** (Potassium bichromate): Sinus pressure and pain. Thick, stringy, yellow-green nasal discharge. Colds that turn into sinus infections.

- *Mercurius* (Mercury): Yellow-green nasal discharge. Foul-smelling breath and sweat. Metallic taste in the mouth. Coated tongue. Feel too hot and too cold.

- **Pulsatilla** (Windflower): "Ripe" cold with thick, bland, yellow-green mucus. Weepy, whiny, clingy, wants affection, company. No thirst. Moods changeable.

PREVENTION

- If exposed: Start taking immune support immediately and frequently in the form of echinacea, olive leaf, ginger, elderberry, garlic, goldenseal, and Vitamins A, C, and zinc. We use the formulas Olive Leaf Relief and Immune-a-Day ourselves, and with our patients.

- Maitake, Reishi, Shitake, and Turkey Tail mushrooms can be effective.

- *Oscillococcinum* (homeopathic remedy from the liver and heart of a wild duck): One dose is often enough for prevention, especially if the cold has a flu-like feeling with it.

- If you are on the edge, rest, avoid being chilled, overstressed, and cut out sugar, caffeine, and alcohol for a few days.

- A saline nasal wash or neti pot can be used to avoid colds.

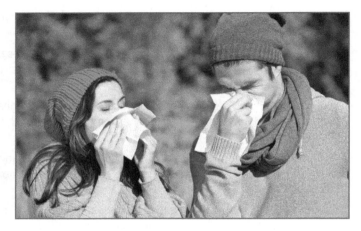

- Don't share water bottles or glasses with your sick travel partners.

MORE NATURAL TIPS

- Drink hot ginger tea with honey and hot lemon juice with honey.

- Avoid dairy products, wheat, bananas, and oatmeal, which cause mucus.

- Pump yourself with the immune support listed above.

- Zinc lozenges can help, especially if you have a sore throat.

- Eat lots of garlic, company permitting, or use garlic capsules.

TRIPSAVERS

- We ALWAYS take our immune support products, keep them handy, and start popping them frequently at the VERY FIRST sign of a cold or flu. www.healthyhomeopathy.com/shop

COLIC

There is nothing like the piercing scream of a miserable infant in the middle of the night to make you the most unpopular parent in your hotel or on the plane! Your bundle of joy may become inconsolable, likely due to gas in the abdomen or stomach. Usually colic passes in a matter of weeks. If your baby does not gain weight, vomits excessively, has persistent diarrhea, or still has symptoms after 6 months of age, seek medical attention.

HOMEOPATHY

- *Calcarea carbonica* (Calcium carbonate): Colic in chubby, stubborn babies who sweat on their heads. Intolerance of mother's milk. Sour burps or vomit.

- *Carbo vegetabilis* (Charcoal): Lots of gas and belching. Relieved by burping the baby. Baby is cold, yet feels better under a fan or from exposure to a draft.

- **Chamomilla** (Chamomile): Screams and cries with the pain. Inconsolable. Wants to be carried or rocked all the time. Fussy. Green, spinach-like diarrhea.

- **Colocynthis** (Bitter cucumber): Agonizing, cutting pain causing the baby to draw the knees to the chest. Better from warmth and from pressure on abdomen. Restless, oversensitive, easily irritated.

- **Lycopodium** (Club moss): Bloating and gas worse 4 to 8PM. Worse from the pressure of diapers or clothing around abdomen. Relieved by warm drinks.

- **Magnesia phosphorica** (Magnesium phosphate): Cramping pain with lots of gas. Relieved by hot applications or drinks, drawing knees to chest, pressure, and rubbing.

- *Nux vomica* (Quaker buttons): Colic with constipation. Arched back and tense muscles. Worse if mother ingests stimulating food/drink. Irritable, impatient.

- *Pulsatilla* (Windflower): Colic in a sweet, clingy, mild baby who fusses, wants to be held and cuddles. Better from fresh air.

PREVENTION

- Moms: Watch what you eat, especially cabbage-family veggies, chocolate, and allergenic foods (dairy, soy, wheat, eggs, corn, and peanuts).

- We advocate giving only or primarily breast milk for the first year, then gradually adding in hypoallergenic foods. If you cannot nurse, we recommend goat's milk. Add 1 t. liquid B vitamins with folic acid to each quart of goat's milk.

- For a specific list of what to introduce, click "Appointment" on our website and scroll down to the list of pdfs: http://healthyhomeopathy.com/appointments/

MORE NATURAL TIPS

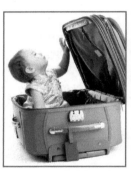

- Burp the baby after eating, and rock or carry to soothe.

- Pacifiers may help with the urge to suck.

- Add ½ t. dill to two cups boiling water. Steep, cool, give 3 times a day.

- A hot water bottle (not too hot) on the abdomen may relieve discomfort.

- Some babies do better if pressure is applied to the tummy.

Honey, I Packed the Baby!

- YouTube has several clear, hands-on videos of moms using various massage and manipulation techniques for their colicky babies.

TRIPSAVERS

- Some moms swear by gripe water, available in most East Indian grocery stores. Dill and sodium bicarbonate are the main ingredients.

CONJUNCTIVITIS (Pink Eye)

Acute inflammation of the thin, protective lining of the eyelids and eyeballs.

HOMEOPATHY

- **Apis** (Honeybee): Eyelids are swollen, puffy, and red. Eyes are bright red, bloodshot. Stinging, burning pains. Hot eyes and tears. Cold compresses help.

- *Argentum nitricum* (Silver nitrate): Conjunctivitis in young children. Eye is red, swollen, pain is splinter-like. Mucus sticks eyelids together.

- *Belladonna* (Deadly nightshade): Comes on suddenly and violently. Red face and fever. Eye is red, hot, light sensitive. Throbbing pains. Worse right eye.

- *Euphrasia* (Eyebright): Eyes water profusely. Hot, irritating tears.

- **Pulsatilla** (Windflower): Profuse, thick, bland, yellow-green discharge. Eyes are stuck together in the morning on waking. Clingy, weepy, and wants comfort, love.

- *Sulphur* (Sulfur): Red, hot, dry, gritty eyes. Burning pain. Yellow, sticky discharge.

PREVENTION

- If exposed, wash hands often with soap and warm water and do NOT touch or rub your eyes. Wash any discharge from eyes several times a day. Clean eyeglasses.

- Do not use someone else's eyedropper bottle or dispenser.

- Wash pillowcases and bedding. Don't share bedding, towels or make-up.

MORE NATURAL TIPS

- Use sterile Eyebright or Boric acid eye drops several times a day in each eye.

- An ice pack can decrease swelling, redness, and itching.

- Dissolve ¼ tsp. salt in one cup of water. Soak cotton balls and swipe the edge of the eyelids from inside to outside 4 times a day, using a fresh cotton ball with each application.

- Vitamin A 25,000 IU/day and Vitamin C 500mg six times a day.

- For allergic conjunctivitis, see ALLERGIC REACTIONS (page 68) and HAY FEVER (page 140).

- In a pinch, apply a mixture of equal parts honey and warm milk with an eyecup, cotton ball, eyedropper, or compress. Keep it sterile.

- Boiled water with dried coriander or fennel, cooled, can be soothing.
- Chamomile teabags make useful, soothing eye pads.

TRIPSAVERS

- Deal with conjunctivitis right away. If left untreated, it may become a recurrent problem or cause serious damage to the eye tissue.

CONSTIPATION

The combination of dehydration, long flights, or periods of time without availability of safe water, beverages, or fruits and vegetables, lack of exercise, lack of availability of clean, private bathrooms, and the general tension and weariness of travel can all predispose one to constipation.

HOMEOPATHY

- **Alumina** (Aluminum): Severe constipation, with no urge for a bowel movement. Dryness of mucus membranes and skin. Stool is so impacted that it must be removed by hand.
- *Bryonia* (Hops): Constipation, together with chapped lips and a dry cough.
- *Calcarea carbonica* (Calcium carbonate): Constipation from low thyroid or in roly-poly infants with large, sweaty heads and flabby bodies.
- **Nux vomica** (Quaker buttons): Constipation with constant urging and terrible straining. Hard, painful stool. Irritable, impatient, competitive people who drive themselves too hard.
- **Silica** (Flint): Bashful stool (comes part way out, then recedes), rabbit pellets. Straining to pass a hard stool.

PREVENTION

- Drink LOTS of water while traveling and eat fresh, juicy, raw food (peeled when appropriate) and eat whole grains and fiber.

- A glass of warm water with lemon on rising can be quite helpful.

- If you tend towards constipation, travel with ground flax seed, and prunes or prune juice, and, if desperate, glycerin rectal suppositories.

- Walk frequently when traveling, whenever and wherever you can.

MORE NATURAL TIPS

- **Judyth:** On my first trip to India in 1981, I discovered psyllium seed husks (Isabgol) to help with both constipation and diarrhea. Drink plenty of water whenever taking psyllium.

- *Triphala* (three fruits) is an Ayurvedic digestive aid.

- Ripe bananas and spicy food can get your gut moving.

- Magnesium citrate 600-800mg/day is a natural alternative to laxatives, as well as being a muscle relaxant.

LIFESAVERS

- A very close friend of ours, normally healthy and stoic, ignored constipation, gas, and bowel pain for two days. She ended up in the hospital with a bowel obstruction. If you need help, get it!

TRIPSAVERS

- Take a healthy, digestive care package including high-fiber protein bars, seeds including flax, dried prunes, psyllium.

- If you have to dump your water before passing through airport security, remember to buy a water bottle before boarding the plane.

- Request a glass of fresh juice, water, or another non-alcoholic beverage whenever it is offered on the plane.

- Walk up and down the aisles during long flights, and do airplane yoga.

COUGHS AND BRONCHITIS

We have found upper and lower respiratory conditions (usually bronchitis) to be a significant travel health challenge, due in large part, to air pollution in urban areas of Third World countries, cigarette smoke pollution in parts of Europe and the Middle East, and, perhaps the worst, contagion on long flights with poor air quality.

Bob: My close call occurred a few days after we flew back from teaching a homeopathic seminar in Europe. On the morning of my 50th birthday party, I began to cough, and felt so terrible that we canceled my party. That night I began to shake. My breathing became rapid. I got up in the middle of the night and coughed up blood into the bathroom sink. The next morning we rushed to the hospital. It was good that we wasted no time. The ER doctor informed us that I would have died within five or six hours from bilateral bacterial pneumonia!

HOMEOPATHY

- *Antimonium tartaricum* (Tartar emetic): Loose, rattling cough without much mucus coming up. Bronchial tubes are full of mucus. Breathing is difficult.

- **Bryonia** (Hops): Dry cough. Dry, chapped mouth and lips. Very thirsty for cold drinks. Everything worse from any movement. Holds the chest while coughing to keep it from moving. Joint pain. Irritable. Homesick.

- *Coccus cacti* (Cochineal): Cough with thick, stringy mucus that causes choking. Constant throat clearing. Racking cough leading to vomiting. Violent tickling.

- **Drosera** (Sundew): Violent fits of hard, dry coughing that end in gagging or vomiting. Barking, croupy, spasmodic cough. Can barely breathe during cough.

- *Ipecacuanha* (Ipecac root, commonly called Ipecac): Vomiting and nausea with loose cough. Nausea not relieved by vomiting. Clear tongue.

- *Pulsatilla* (Windflower): Bronchitis with thick yellow or green nasal discharge and expectoration. Weepy, whiny, clingy, wants

C

affection and company. No thirst. Moody. Symptoms are worse in a hot, stuffy room.

- **Rumex** (Yellow dock): Dry cough from a tickle in the throat near the Adam's apple. Cough is worse from uncovering the body or getting undressed.

- **Spongia** (Toasted sponge): Dry, barking, suffocating cough. Like a saw cutting through wood or a seal barking. Cough better after eating or drinking. Croup.

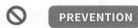

PREVENTION

- If you feel on the edge of an upper respiratory infection while traveling, try, if at all possible, to lay low for a day or two, until you recover.

- If your travel partner has a cough and a cold, protect yourself with rest, and immune support. Don't share eating utensils, and, if possible, sleep in another room. Ask him or her to cover nose and mouth while sneezing or coughing and to dispose of used tissues.

- If you suffer from asthma or other chronic lung problems, consider receiving constitutional treatment from a homeopath before you leave. If that is not an option, visit your doctor well before you leave for a checkup and a medication refill.

- If visiting an urban area known for its severe pollution, such as Mumbai, Tokyo, Taiwan, Kathmandu, Mexico City, or Manila, take a mask, or at least a handkerchief, to cover your nose and mouth.

- Research hotels and restaurants ahead of time to avoid smokers. Sit indoors in non-smoking restaurants rather than outdoors with smokers.

- Choose bus or train seats next to windows that open. For local trips, sitting near the driver may allow more fresh air from the opening door, especially if the windows do not open.

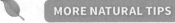

MORE NATURAL TIPS

- For wet coughs: hot ginger tea with honey or lemon juice with honey. Lemon juice helps cut mucus.

- Licorice root tea is also effective in bringing up mucus.
- We use Sitopaladi, an Ayurvedic powdered mixture with heating herbs, including cinnamon, cardamom, long pepper and bamboo in a rock candy base. You may find it at Indian stores.
- Wild cherry bark cough syrup: ½ tsp. up to 6 times a day. When using homeopathy, avoid eucalyptus, pine, camphor, and menthol products.
- Take Vitamin C 500mg, and Vitamin A 5,000 IU every four hours.
- Suck zinc lozenges or take zinc 30mg/day.
- Avoid dairy products, sweets, caffeine, alcohol, and heavy foods.
- Drink herb teas and fresh carrot and other veggie and fruit juices.

 LIFESAVERS

- If you have a persistent, exhausting cough with chest pain and weakness, have a check up to make sure it is not pneumonia, TB, or some other serious contagious disease.

 TRIPSAVERS

- We always take with us immune support (especially Immune-a-Day and Olive Leaf Relief), wherever and whenever we travel. At the VERY first sign of a scratchy throat, cough, or flu, we start taking them every two hours. Whichever your immune boosters of choice, take them immediately and frequently. Often, after a couple of days, you will be symptom-free and good to go.
- **Judyth:** I can sometimes catch a cold from exposure to cigarette smoke, so I take a small, battery-operated fan for emergencies.

CUTS, SCRAPES, AND PUNCTURE WOUNDS

For minor wounds: apply direct pressure to stop bleeding and clean the wound with soap and water, 3% hydrogen peroxide (one part peroxide to 9 parts water), *Calendula* tincture diluted with water (1:1), or an iodine preparation. Cover the wound with a bandage or gauze dressing and change frequently. Superficial wounds are not serious and generally heal quickly on their own, if kept clean and free of infection. However, a minor scrape that you would not bat an eyelash over in first-world countries can take on a different level of magnitude in a country where cleanliness is not the norm, AIDS and other infectious diseases are widespread, the blood quality for transfusions is not trustworthy, and quality medical care may be hours or days away.

For severe bleeding: apply direct pressure on the wound. Soak puncture wounds in warm water several times a day to remove additional debris. Deep cuts or puncture wounds may need stitches and require immediate medical attention, as will serious wounds, such as from a knife or gunshot.

Bob: I whacked my head on a slow-moving ceiling fan in Puerto Escondido, Mexico while standing on the bed to move the curtains in order to improve our ocean view. Ouch! A dose of *Arnica*, and some ice cubes in a washcloth, led to a speedy recovery. The view improved, too!

HOMEOPATHY

- *Arnica* (Leopard's bane): Any trauma or wound with bruising or bleeding. Shock.

- *Hypericum* (St. John's wort): Cuts or injuries to nerve-rich areas, such as the tips of fingers and toes. Shooting pains. Numbness and tingling.

- *Ledum* (Marsh tea): Puncture wounds that are cold to the touch and better from ice or cold applications. Use with tetanus immunization.

PREVENTION

- A tetanus booster is recommended every ten years after your initial vaccination.

MORE NATURAL TIPS

- Apply *Calendula* gel, cream, spray (abrasions) or tincture (1:3 with water). If available, add *Hypericum* tincture to prevent infection.

- Apply colloidal silver spray topically.

- For general wound healing: Vitamin C 500mg four times/day, zinc 30mg/day, and Vitamin A 25,000 IU/day.

- Echinacea and goldenseal tincture 30 drops three times a day in water or juice to fight infection and stimulate the immune system.

- Don't put topical *Arnica* on broken skin—it can cause a rash. Save it for bruises.

LIFESAVERS

- Puncture wounds carry the risk of tetanus within two days to two months after the wound has become infected. Early signs of tetanus include jaw stiffness, difficulty swallowing, and stiffness of the neck, arms, or legs following a puncture wound. Tetanus shots are 100% effective in preventing tetanus. Though tetanus infections are very rare, the death rate is about 25%, greater if over 50. If you have not kept up on the tetanus boosters or have low immunity, TIG (tetanus immune globulin) may be recommended. It starts working quickly. If you have any kind of wound deep enough for oxygen to not be present, even surgery, it is a good idea to get a tetanus booster, if you have not done so within the past ten years. The tetanus booster is generally given as a Tdap (tetanus, diphtheria, and pertussis) combination. The new Tdap does not contain thimerosal (mercury preservative). Some physicians *do* offer tetanus-only boosters.

DEEP VEIN THROMBOSIS (DVT; Tourist/Economy-Class Syndrome)

DVT is a blood clot in a deep vein, predominantly in the legs. Symptoms include pain, heat, redness, swelling, and engorged superficial veins. It is not that common (affecting about one in 1000 adults) but it can result in a pulmonary embolism, which may be life threatening, and long haul air travel is a predisposing factor. Most cases in travelers occur along with one of the other risk factors, which include pregnancy, use of estrogen medication (in the form of hormone replacement or birth control pills), obesity, smoking, varicose veins, previous history of DVT or pulmonary embolus, recent injury or surgery, age over 60, or chronic disease such as heart disease or cancer. DVT was first reported in 1940 in London in the underground railway stations during extended air raids, and can also be aggravated by long travel on crowded buses or cars.

HOMEOPATHY

- **Hamamelis** (Witch hazel): Varicose veins; soreness, bruising, swelling, or hemorrhages of or from veins. Worse touch.

- **Secale** (Ergot of rye): DVT after surgery.

PREVENTION

- Wear comfortable, loose-fitting clothing.

- It is wise for those at increased risk to wear below-the-knee elastic, graduated-compression stockings.

- Avoid crossing the legs at the ankles or knees. Walk up and down the aisles and stretch. Change leg position often. Wiggle your toes and legs while in your seat. Walk in airports and elevate your legs when you can.

- Here are a few in-flight exercises suggested by American Airlines. Do not do them if contraindicated by your doctor or if they cause pain:
    1. Ankle circles: Lift your foot off the floor and draw a circle in the air with toes pointed, alternating directions. Continue for 30 seconds. Repeat with the other foot.
    2. Foot pumps: Keep your heels on the floor and point feet up as high as possible toward the head. Lower both feet back flat on the floor. Keep balls of feet on floor while lifting both heels high. Continue for 30 seconds.
    3. Knee lifts: While seated, march slowly in place by contracting one thigh muscle, then the other. Continue for 30 seconds.

4. Knee to chest: Hold your left knee, pulling up toward the chest for 10 to 15 seconds. Slowly return to floor. Alternate legs 10 times.

- Request an exit row seat or, at least, an aisle seat, so it will be easy to exit your row without climbing over seatmates.

- If at risk, it might be worth researching the configuration of plane choices before booking, since the amount of legroom varies considerably.

- If your risk is very high, consider alternative forms of transportation.

- Drink lots of water, rather than alcohol and coffee, to prevent dehydration. We take our favorite herb tea bags with us when we fly.

- For those at risk, take an aspirin, with food, four hours before the flight.

MORE NATURAL TIPS

- *Capsella bursa* (Butcher's broom) is an herbal remedy helpful for varicose veins.

- Omega-3 fish oil, Arginine (we use a Thorne Research product called Perfusia SR), Co-Q 50 or 100, and Vitamin E 200-600 IU can be supportive of a healthy bloodstream.

- Equal parts lemon and baking soda, to alkalinize the system may help.

LIFESAVERS

- If you are at risk and you become aware of the symptoms mentioned above during your travels, find a reputable doctor and consider changing your return travel plans.

DENGUE FEVER

Dengue fever is a viral infection transmitted by the *Aedes aegypti* mosquito. In recent years, it has made a comeback, due to the population increases in urban areas, poverty, and global warming. It is endemic in more than 100 countries and infects about 50 million people each year. Since these bugs breed in small accumulations of water, such as empty tires, cans, planters, they can be a problem for tourists, especially during or after the rainy season in tropical areas. Symptoms are: first a high fever, severe headache behind the eyes, and intense bone pain (it is called "breakbone" or "bonecrusher" fever.) There may be a rash on day four or five. It usually gets better on its own after a week, but fatigue and aching may persist. It may be confused with malaria.

HOMEOPATHY

- *China* (Peruvian bark): Periodic fevers with exhaustion, weakness, and headache. Perspiration day and night, during sleep. Bloating, gas.

- **Eupatorium perfoliatum** (Boneset): Most often the correct remedy for dengue. Fevers with pain as if the bones were broken. Aching or bruised feeling deep in bones. Restless. Very thirsty. Painful soreness of the eyeballs. Scanty perspiration.

- *Gelsemium* (Yellow jasmine): Dizzy, drowsy, droopy and dull. Flu-like exhaustion. Chills up back. Not thirsty.

- *Tabacum* (Tobacco): Severe nausea, dizziness, abdominal and leg cramps. Heart palpitations. Extreme chilliness.

PREVENTION

- There is no vaccine and no effective conventional treatment, so preventing spread by the mosquito is key. Mosquito coils and electric mosquito mats   placed near entrances can be a stopgap measure, but may prove deleterious to human health over time. www.ecademy.com/node.php?id=62727

- Spray your outer clothing with permethrin (or soak) before your trip and use repellant (preferably 10% or less DEET) for hands, face, and other exposed areas.

- Wear long-sleeved shirts, long pants, and socks.

- Cover beds with mosquito netting and tuck it in. Or find a room with AC.

MORE NATURAL TIPS

- We have not treated dengue fever, but came across a recommendation by a Brazilian homeopath for a combination of the following medicines:

- *China* (Peruvian bark), *Gelsemium* (Yellow jasmine), *Eupatorium perfoliatum* (Bonset), *Ledum* (Marsh tea), and *Rhus tox.* (Poison ivy). If the single medicines that we list are not working, or if you prefer to play it safe and have the combo, it makes sense to us. It should be available through any homeopathic pharmacy. Take every two hours at onset of dengue, then every 3 or 4 hours until symptoms go away. Can be given to babies, pregnant moms, and used preventively. www.naturalhealthstrategies.com/dengue-fever.html

LIFESAVERS

- Dengue hemorrhagic fever (not covered here) can be fatal. It occurs when one catches a second, different type of dengue virus. Fortunately, only a small number of the over 100 million cases of dengue fever annually develop into dengue hemorrhagic fever. It is possible, though not common, for a traveler returning to the U.S. with a dengue infection to pass it on to someone who has not traveled. Those under 12, female, and Caucasian are more susceptible. Early symptoms, similar to those of dengue fever, are: fever, headaches, appetite loss, joint aches, malaise, muscle aching, vomiting. This is followed by restlessness and sweating, then bruising; a rash all over the body; and small red spots on the skin. This progresses to sweating, cold and clammy extremities, and shock. Hospitalization is essential. There is no known cure or vaccine for Dengue hemorrhagic fever. If *any* of these symptoms occur, seek immediate emergency care.

TRIPSAVERS

- Carry a good-quality mosquito net when visiting tropical areas in rainy season, especially in Central and South America, India and SE Asia.

DIARRHEA (See Also Cholera, Food Poisoning, Typhoid)

Traveler's diarrhea, a.k.a. Montezuma's revenge, Delhi belly, Karachi crouch, Turista, the Aztec Two-Step, and Turkey trots, is the most common health problem affecting travelers—up to ten million per year. Commonly accompanied by abdominal cramps, bloating, and nausea, it can put you out of commission fast, and turn your destination of choice into the nearest bathroom. High-risk areas include developing countries in Asia, Africa, the Middle East, and Latin America. The cause is generally a bug: *E. coli, Campylobacter, Shigella,* or *Salmonella* being the most common bacteria. Amebic dysentery is a parasitic infection caused by the *Entamoeba histolytica* amoeba. *Giardia lamblia* is a protozoan. They are introduced into your system when you drink impure water or eat contaminated food, causing watery stools, abdominal cramping, nausea, appetite loss, gas, and mild to severe dehydration.

These differential tips may help you sort out what is the cause:

- Amebic dysentery—One to several weeks after being infected. Abdominal cramps and bloody diarrhea.

- Food poisoning—Vomiting (and sometimes diarrhea, cramping) begins soon after eating and the episode is over within 24 to 48 hours.

- *Giardia* infection—Sudden onset of explosive diarrhea; abdominal cramping, bloating, gas. Symptoms start 2 to 6 weeks after infection.

- Irritable bowel syndrome (IBS)—Alternating diarrhea and constipation, cramping. Chronic problem may begin after acute traveler's diarrhea.

- *Shigella* dysentery—Fever, bloody stool, bad cramps beginning 2 to 3 days after infection.

- Traveler's diarrhea—Diarrhea with some bloating, gas. Starts within several days of your arrival.

We have had our share of the runs, especially given our numerous trips to India. We have successfully treated many patients, as well as our dogs, for diarrhea.

Judyth: While on a 6-day trek on the Milford Track in New Zealand, I resisted the temptation of drinking out of the ubiquitous waterfalls and streams, mostly out of habit since the guide assured us they were pure, and free of *Giardia*. Near the end of the trail, I gave in. A week or two after being back, I developed explosive diarrhea. One dose of *Podophyllum* was all that I needed. The same story with our dear golden retriever, Truffle, after she was diagnosed with *Giardia* for her bleeding stools. One dose did the trick.

HOMEOPATHY

- *Aloe* (Aloe socotrina): Lumpy, slimy, jelly-like, mucous, watery stools that slide out without urging. May be bright yellow. Rectal burning after bowel movement.

- **Arsenicum album** (Arsenic): Severe abdominal cramping, burning pains rectum and abdomen. Diarrhea after bad food, especially meat. Nausea and vomiting after eating or drinking. Very anxious and restless. Waking after midnight. Cold. Desire for frequent sips of water.

- *Chamomilla* (Chamomile): Chopped-spinach-like diarrhea that smells like rotten eggs in fussy children with accompanying fever and/or teething pain.

- *China* (Peruvian bark): Exhausting, cyclic abdominal bloating with frequent belching, which does not help. Feel as if all the blood were drained out. Best medicine for exhaustion after loss of fluids in general.

- *Croton tiglium* (Croton oil seed): Diarrhea gushing out, like a fire hydrant. Worse right after eating or drinking. Gurgling in intestines from eating or drinking the least amount. Sloshing in gut. May be accompanied with a rash.

- *Gambogia* (Gummi gutti tree): Severe diarrhea that gushes out suddenly. Stool comes out in thin, prolonged gushes.

- **Podophyllum** (May apple): #1 medicine in many cases. Urgent, gushing, exhausting diarrhea shooting all over the toilet. Abdominal cramping, rumbling, and gurgling before stool or painless diarrhea. Driven out of bed at 5AM to toilet.

- **Sulphur** (Sulfur): Sudden, smelly, explosive diarrhea drives her out of bed at 5AM. (*Podophyllum*) Hot, rashes, sticks feet out from under covers. Likes sweets, not fish. Anus is itchy, red, sore, raw, burning.

- **Veratrum album** (White hellebore): Violent diarrhea and vomiting with cold sweats. Icy cold. Strong craving for ice, cold drinks, juicy fruits, sour, salty.

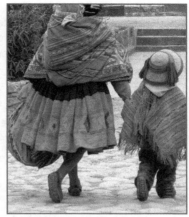

Manta (shawl) baby pack in Sacred Valley, Peru

 PREVENTION

- Wash your hands often with soap and water. Pack an antibacterial gel, or alcohol wipes, and keep them handy.

- Be careful to not drink out of taps in questionable areas, and not even to ingest ice cubes! Water is safe pretty much everywhere in Chile, for example, but not in Peru and Bolivia.

- In some countries, like India, rumor has it that even bottled water comes right out of the tap. If you are back in the bush, do your research, boil water, if needed, take a state-of-the-art ultraviolet pen water filter, or, as awful as they taste, iodine or chlorine pills (buffered Vitamin C helps mask the taste).

- We have been at group retreats in India where food is served en masse, and there is neither a dishwasher nor hot water to wash dishes and utensils. At the very least, a rinse with a bit of bleach will help sanitize and cut down the transmission of contagious disease.

- Peel fruits and veggies before eating.

- Raw seafood and milk products can be high-risk for bacterial contamination.

- Much cooked street food, worldwide, is safe, tasty, and cheap (though often greasy). We ate, not long ago, at the Otavalo, Ecuador market where cooking and cleaning facilities were basic. We stuck to rice, potatoes, cooked beets, and eggs, and were fine.

MORE NATURAL TIPS

- The BRAT diet (bananas, rice, and toast), supplemented with bland veggie soup and applesauce (the pectin helps with diarrhea) or even apples, is reliable for diarrhea. Crackers can substitute for toast.

- Pushing LOTS of fluid (water and electrolyte-rich drinks containing sodium and potassium) is essential to counteract the fluid loss from diarrhea. Even more so if you are vomiting as well. Recharge, Emergen-C, salty vegetable broths, or whatever natural electrolyte replacement you can find locally should work. Pedialyte, if necessary, for infants, to supplement breast milk. For children: starches, cereals, yogurt, fruits, and vegetables.

- Psyllium-seed products (*Isabgol* in India) can help. Lots of water while using these to avoid bloating. (A friend loaded up on psyllium with little water and was painfully bloated for days.) Drink at least 6 glasses of water a day for every teaspoon of psyllium.

- A warm pack over the abdomen or castor oil pack with a heating pad may reduce pain and discomfort.

- In a pinch, charcoal absorbs gas (take capsules or even burnt toast).

- Calcium 1000mg and Magnesium 500mg may relieve cramping.

- Some folks swear by adding a little cider vinegar to their drinking water to strengthen their digestive immunity.

LIFESAVERS

- Do NOT drink cold drinks from a street vendor's stall where flies can transmit bacteria and hygiene is nonexistent. If you hang around a bit, you may notice that the wash or rinse water is far from appetizing, much less hygienic. Boiled drinks, such as chai tea, is fine.

- If your severe diarrhea persists, especially with fever, dehydration, and bloody diarrhea, get medical attention to rule out something serious, like typhoid. Do NOT let yourself get dehydrated, especially if you are out in the boonies. You do not want to end up on IV fluids in a primitive hospital with unsterile needles, and a high incidence of HIV. Heads up: babies and the elderly people can die very quickly of dehydration.

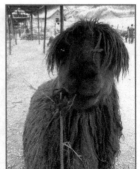
Vegan. Pisaq, Peru

TRIPSAVERS

• Go bland! During our previous, frequent trips to India, we invariably ended up with diarrhea from all the spicy food 24/7 (even breakfast). Two to three weeks into the trip, we found ourselves subsisting on rice, yogurt, and chapattis. It only took a few days for our guts to recover.

DIZZINESS (See Also Motion Sickness)

Dizziness, or vertigo can be caused by something as minor as flu, intoxication from chemical fumes, an acute, incapacitating hangover, or an inner ear infection (labyrinthitis). It may also be the symptom of a more serious condition such as a brain tumor or a stroke or a chronic disease like Ménière's Disease or Multiple Sclerosis.

HOMEOPATHY

• *Aconite* (Monkshood): Sudden dizziness from fright or shock. Vertigo with panic attacks, claustrophobia. Extreme anxiety and restlessness. Profuse sweating. Fear of death, or predicts the time of death.

• *Bryonia* (Hops): Dizziness worse from any motion, getting up from a seat or a bed, turning the head, or bending forward. Dry mouth and lips with extreme thirst. Very irritable. Wants to go home.

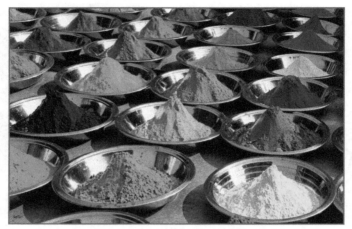

Colorful tica powders in Orcha market, India

- **Cocculus** (Indian cockle): Dizziness due to motion sickness or from looking at moving objects out of a window. Vertigo after losing sleep, especially when caring for an ill family member. Room spins. Must lie down. Headache, nausea, vomiting with the vertigo.

- **Conium** (Poison hemlock): Dizziness worse lying in bed or turning over in bed. Worse moving eyes or head. Feels like the room is spinning.

- **Gelsemium** (Yellow jasmine): Dizzy, drowsy, droopy, and dull with flu. Vertigo from stage fright. Muscle aches, dull mind, blurred vision, heavy eyelids.

- *Pulsatilla* (Windflower): Dizziness from being in a warm, stuffy room. Worse sitting and looking upward; better from walking, lying down, or fresh air. Weepy, moody, clingy, wants company and affection. Lack of thirst.

🚫 **PREVENTION**

- If your balance is compromised, use precautions like taking a cane, walker, or special clips for your shoes if you will be walking on ice.

- If you have Ménière's disease, limit dietary salt.

- If you are at risk for a stroke, stop smoking, eat light, healthy foods, exercise, cut out alcohol, and monitor your blood pressure and cholesterol.

- Avoid high-risk travel activities such as hiking on muddy, slippery, narrow, or precipitous trails, paragliding, bungee jumping, ziplining, wingsuit flying, or rock climbing if you are prone to vertigo or falling.

- Get help, if needed, carrying heavy luggage.

 MORE NATURAL TIPS

- Sit down and close your eyes.

- Pick a point and look at it to regain orientation and balance.

 PREVENTION

- If you begin to feel dizzy, hold on to something secure to prevent falling. Do not drive or operate machinery.

- If you are kayaking or operating a boat, let someone else take over.

- If you find yourself in a terrifyingly unsafe situation where you are at risk of falling, bow out, even at the risk of embarrassment.

EAR INFECTIONS

Infants and young children are particularly prone to acute middle ear infections (otitis media). The pain of an ear infection can be sudden, intense, and intolerable—so much so that we will interrupt our patient schedule if a patient calls suffering from an ear infection. Infections may be internal or external, in the ear canal outside or inside the eardrum. Symptoms include acute pain, a clogged sensation, temporary loss of hearing, and redness and bulging of the eardrum. At times the eardrum can rupture, discharging pus and fluid into the ear canal. Do not worry if it does rupture: it is releasing pressure, and will usually rapidly heal itself. But do NOT put any drops in the ear if the eardrum has burst.

> ### Do Your Gut a Favor
>
> Unsweetened, preferably natural, live yogurt will replenish the healthy flora in your intestine. This is essential after taking antibiotics. We use a *Saccharomyces boulardii* product with our patients—the only probiotic we know of that is antibiotic-resistant and can be taken during a course of antibiotics (also needs no refrigeration, so handy for travel).

HOMEOPATHY

- ***Aconite*** (Monkshood): Sudden onset of an ear infection, worse after being exposed to a cold, dry wind. Very painful, high fever, usually only give within first 24 hours. Ears bright red. Very noise-sensitive. Fearful, restless.

- ***Belladonna*** (Deadly nightshade): Sudden, violent ear infections, especially the right ear. Bright red face, high fever, glassy eyes. Intense, throbbing pain. Sensitive to light, noise, jarring. Throbbing headache. Better dark room.

- ***Chamomilla*** (Chamomile): Great pain with red-hot ears. Can occur during teething. Hypersensitive to and inconsolable with the pain. Can't bear to be touched. Child is very irritable. Demands to be held or carried.

- *Hepar sulphuris* (Calcium sulfide): Ears very painful. Thick pus behind eardrum with bad-smelling or sour-smelling discharge. Can't bear to be touched. Child wakes screaming. Very cold. Oversensitive, annoyed.

- *Mercurius* (Mercury): Sharp or stinging pain in the ears. Discharge of bad-smelling, yellow-green pus or thin, bloody discharge. Salivation or drooling. Bad breath and foul smelling sweat. Sensitive to heat and cold. Worse at night.

- **Pulsatilla** (Windflower): Ears feel stopped up. Thick, bland yellow-green discharge from nose, ears, lungs. A ripe cold with profuse, thick nasal discharge. Ears ache at night. Clingy, weepy, wants fresh air. Not thirsty.

- **Silica** (Flint): Chronic ear infections. Eardrum can rupture. Ear is filled with bad smelling pus. Swollen lymph nodes, low energy, smelly feet.

E

PREVENTION

- The most common cause of otitis media in infants is being introduced too early to cow's milk or formula. We recommend breast milk and, if supplementation is necessary, goat's milk.

- Wear a hat or earmuffs if playing out in cold weather.

- Remove allergens from the diet (consider dairy, wheat, corn). We have found cow's milk dairy to be the worst. Alternatives are hazelnut, goat, sheep, and even camel, milk.

- Vitamin A 25,000 IU (2,000 IU infant) and Vitamin C 2,000 mg (500mg infant) for acute cases of otitis media.

- For infants: Never prop up a bottle while feeding an infant. Hold upright while feeding or place the head significantly higher so that the milk will not drain into the Eustachian tube. Do not give an infant a bottle while lying in bed (milk can pool in middle ear). Better to breastfeed!

- Stay away from first- and second-hand cigarette and cigar smoke.

- If your child is highly environmentally allergic, consider a HEPA filter to remove allergens from the air.

- Monitor your small child for any sign of hearing loss.

- Teach your child to blow his or her nose properly.

MORE NATURAL TIPS

- Place warm mullein-garlic ear drops in the affected ear three times a day. Warm bottle or dropper under faucet first. A piece of cotton in the ear will prevent the oil from coming out. If there is a tendency to infection in both ears, place the drops in both.

- Alternating hot (3 minutes) and cold compresses (1 minute) to the affected ear. Or have the child lie with the ear on a warmed towel.

 LIFESAVERS

- For an ear infection with a fever over 103F and severe pain that does not resolve, consult a pediatrician to rule out mastoiditis.

- If there is a violent headache with the ear pain and it is excruciating to bend the head forward touching chin to neck, consult with a pediatrician to rule out meningitis.

✈ **TRIPSAVERS**

- If your small child begins to pull or tug on the ears, develops a fever, cries without cause, or shakes the head repeatedly, check for otitis.

- If you cannot find herbal eardrops, you can make your own from olive oil and garlic. Apply warm, as indicated above.

- If you suspect an ear infection, begin treatment immediately. Studies, and our clinical experience, indicate that antibiotic treatment does not result in a long-term cure for otitis media. We have found homeopathy very effective for the immediate infection and for long-term prevention.

FAINTING

This sudden, brief loss of consciousness, due to a lowering of blood pressure to the brain, may result from physical causes such as blood loss, dehydration, pain, becoming overheated, exhaustion, overexertion, hyperventilation, or heart arrhythmias. Emotional causes include panic, fright, and shock. Fainting is a medical emergency until proven otherwise. It is vital to rule out trauma, injury, heart attack, stroke, or other emergency before moving the person.

HOMEOPATHY

- *Aconite* (Monkshood): Fainting from fear, fright, or anxiety. Can be sudden. Fears impending death. Extreme restlessness. Rapid pulse. Violent heart palpitations. Profuse sweating. Fears crowds, airplanes, earthquakes.

- ***Arnica*** (Leopard's bane): Fainting from blood loss, shock, after an accident or traumatic injury. Trauma, injuries, falls, sprains, strains. Bleeding anywhere in the body. Bruising. Says nothing is wrong and refuses help.

- ***Carbo vegetabilis*** (Charcoal): Acute episodes of fainting. Collapsed, weak, exhausted with difficulty breathing. Wants to be fanned. Fainting from indigestion, loss of body fluids. Gas and belching. Pale. Bluish skin. Very cold.

- *China* (Peruvian bark): Fainting from loss of bodily fluids, especially blood loss. Periodic fever with chills, weakness, drenching sweats, and exhaustion.

- *Coffea* (Unroasted coffee): Fainting from joy, excitement, pain. Oversensitive.

- *Gelsemium* (Yellow jasmine): Fainting from stage fright. Performance anxiety.

- *Ignatia* (St. Ignatius bean): Fainting from grief, profound grief or disappointment. Uncontrollable sobbing. Frequent sighing. Lump in the throat. Chest tight.

- *Veratrum album* (White hellebore): Collapse after vomiting, diarrhea. Fainting after BM, vomiting, bleeding. Face bluish. Icy cold. Profuse sweat. Wants ice and cold drinks, juicy fruit, sour, and salty. Restless and busy.

PREVENTION

- If you feel faint, lie down.
- Be aware of and deal with underlying medical problems.
- Carefully evaluate prescription medications for side effects.

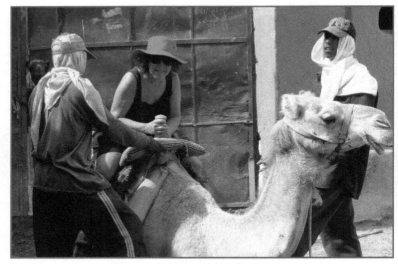

Hold on and don't faint!

- Learn stress management techniques if you faint for emotional reasons.

MORE NATURAL TIPS

- Moisten the lips or tongue with a few drops of Bach Flower Essence Rescue Remedy.

- Apply a cold washcloth to the forehead.

- Place a handkerchief with three drops of peppermint oil over the nose.

- Herbal *Gingko biloba* 40-80mg may help increase and improve blood circulation to the brain. May be contraindicated if you are taking anticonvulsants, antidepressants, or blood-thinning or blood pressure medications.

- Bilberry, a relative of blueberry, has been shown to improve circulation.

LIFESAVERS

- Have the person lie down. If it is not possible to lie down, sit with your head between your knees. If you suspect someone is about to faint, help them lie down. If a person faints and does not regain consciousness within 1-2 minutes, put them into the recovery position by placing on the side supported by one arm and one leg. Then do the following:

  - Check to make sure airway is clear.

  - Check breathing and pulse. Begin CPR if necessary.

  - Loosen clothing, belts, and collar.

  - Elevate feet above head.

  - If patient is not normal within one minute, seek medical help.

 TRIPSAVERS

- We were on an express train in India from Pune to Mumbai. The older gentleman in the row in front of us, who was traveling with his daughter, appeared to faint. We could see from behind that, after quickly reviving, he requested the overhead fan to be directed towards him. We gave him a dose of *Carbo vegetabilis*. He perked up almost immediately, but the conductor had already been alerted, which set in motion a bureaucratic procedure, as is typical in India. The man needed no further medical attention (the fan remained on). Homeopathy was the unsung hero.

FEAR OF FLYING

Aviophobia, fear of flying, may be related exclusively to air travel, or may be related to other fears such as claustrophobia (fear of enclosed spaces), agoraphobia (fear of going out in public, especially when they cannot escape), acrophobia (fear of heights), or a fear of vomiting, terrorist attack, impending death, drowning, or simply a loss of control. Nearly three million passengers fly every day worldwide. It is estimated that 1/3 to 1/2 of the population suffers from fear of flying at least once in their lives. **Judyth:** Intense fear of flying may lead to a panic attack, which I experienced first-hand. I was flying to a homeopathic conference in Minneapolis a little over twenty years ago. It was a sweltering summer day, and my flight was stuck on the runway for an hour. Next to me, spilling over onto my seat, sat an obese woman. For the first time in my life, I began to experience a panic attack: shortness of breath, rapid heartbeat, and anxiety. When the symptoms became even more intense, I alerted a crewmember. Believe it or not, the pilot turned around the plane and dropped me off at the departure gate *with* my checked bag. I received and filled a prescription for Xanax, which I never used. Although I have never again experienced anything to that degree, I did, for a period of time, fear that I *might*. When I flew alone a year ago from Chile to Germany to Egypt, Bob was kind enough to record a 10-minute relaxation exercise for me on iTunes. Fortunately I didn't even *think* about using it. We met a woman recently who actually persuaded pilots to turn the plane around for her THREE times!"

HOMEOPATHY

- **Aconite** (Monkshood): Fear of planes and crowds. Sudden fright and emotional shock about the flight. Terrified of impending death. Great anxiety and restlessness. Rapid heartbeat. Violent palpitations. Profuse sweating.

- **Argentum nitricum** (Silver nitrate): Anticipatory anxiety and apprehension before the flight. Fear of heights, being trapped. Worried about making the flight on time. Impulse to jump out of the plane. Fear of elevators and bridges.

- *Arsenicum album* (Arsenic): Tremendous pre-flight anxiety. Fear of dying when the plane crashes. Extreme worry about health. Insomnia after midnight. Cold.

- *Calcarea carbonica* (Calcium carbonate): Anxiety about safety and natural disasters in general: fear of flying, heights, earthquakes, storms, security, mice. May be overweight, flabby. Calf cramps. Sweat on scalp. Loves eggs.

PREVENTION

- Watch YouTube videos and other free online courses to free you of your fear.

- Take the indicated homeopathic medicine four hours before your flight.

- Allow plenty of time to travel to the airport, check in, proceed through security, and even have a meal or a snack, if that relaxes you.

- Treat yourself to an airport seated chair massage just prior to your flight. You deserve it!

- Pack lightly so you have less to worry about. If you check baggage, label it well and make it a different color than black so it will stand out. If you do need to put carry-on luggage overhead, try to board early so that it will be less stressful.

- If you are traveling to a new destination, bring a travel book to keep you busy until you arrive.

- If it makes you feel better, research the safety, on-time arrivals, and seating configuration of the plane alternatives and choose what puts you most at ease. www.seatguru.com

- Know what to expect, understand why flying is normally safe, sit in a wing seat, and breathe fresh air.

- Have your travel documents and money organized and easily accessible so you will not need to worry about them.

MORE NATURAL TIPS

- Try out airplane yoga. www.airplaneyoga.com

- Deep breathing exercises, even without the yoga, are very relaxing. Close your eyes and breathe in and out slowly through both nostrils, do alternate nostril breathing, or inhale and exhale only through the left nostril (a calming breath).

- Skip the alcohol and caffeine, drink plenty of water, and eat as healthily as possible on the plane. Becoming hypoglycemic or dehydrated will only make you more anxious. Take along healthy, delicious food or snacks.

 LIFESAVERS

- Though not a matter of life and death, plane anxiety may feel that way at the time. Remember, you can always get a prescription for a mild sedative such as Xanax. It may be enough to only keep it in your pocket, knowing that you have it, just in case!

 TRIPSAVERS

- Organize beforehand your travel toiletries to satisfy the U.S. Transportation Security Agency or TSA and to decrease last-minute stress.

- Take Rescue Remedy as often as needed during the flight.

- Bring engaging reading materials, either in book, e-book, or magazine, to occupy your attention.

- Book an aisle or exit row seat in order to have more legroom and ability to get up and walk around during the flight.

- Travel with a buddy. If alone, strike up a conversation with your seatmate(s). You may or may not want to share with them that you are nervous, depending on who they are and what makes you feel best.

- Make a personal connection with the flight attendants so you feel they are on your team.

- On long flights, watch entertaining, non-suspenseful movies to pass the time more quickly.

- Bring along a recorded deep-relaxation tape or music tape, either standard or recorded just for you, to relax mind and spirit.

- Meditate, sing to yourself, or sleep— whatever is most calming.

F

FEVER

Fever is a natural mechanism of the body to respond to disease and bring you back into balance. It is when fevers are high (above 104F /40C) that there can be a problem. Chills often precede or accompany a fever, and sweats occur when the fever is breaking.

HOMEOPATHY

- **Aconite** (Monkshood): High fevers that come on suddenly and violently. Fevers after a shock, fright, or exposure to a cold, dry wind. Sudden dry, croupy cough. Dry skin, mouth. Contracted pupils. Violent heart palpitations. Rapid pulse. Profuse perspiration. Anxiety.

- **Belladonna** (Deadly nightshade): Fevers come on suddenly and violently. Bright-red, flushed face, fever above 103F/39.4C. Very red, sore throat. Right-sided. Highly sensitive to light, noise, jar. Dilated pupils. Desire for lemons or lemon drinks.

- *Chamomilla* (Chamomile): Childhood fever due to ear infections or teething. Extremely pain sensitive. Screams, arches back, inconsolable.

- *China* (Peruvian bark): Periodic fevers with chills, weakness, drenching sweats, and exhaustion. Loss of bodily fluids (blood, diarrhea, or excessive perspiration). Fever rises and falls, as though on a schedule.

- *Ferrum phosphoricum* (Iron phosphate): High fever with flushed face, especially round, red spots on cheeks. First stage of a nondescript acute illness where fever is the prominent symptom.

- *Pulsatilla* (Windflower): Fevers in children who are weepy, clingy, moody. Hot in a warm, stuffy room. Better fresh air. Little thirst.

PREVENTION

- Sun protection can prevent a fever due to overexposure.

- Following sound hygiene may protect you from contracting fevers due to contagious diseases.

- If at risk for a fever, we recommend immune boosting products containing echinacea, elderberry, goldenseal, Vitamin A, C, and E.

MORE NATURAL TIPS

- Drink plenty of fluids to counteract fluid loss through perspiration.

- We recommend the cold, wet sock treatment to break a fever. Take a hot shower or soak in a hot bathtub. Drink hot sage or yarrow tea. Put cold, wet socks on your feet and cover with plastic bags. Bundle up in warm blankets. Go to bed. Your fever should break during the night.

- Take a tepid sponge bath with water or diluted apple cider vinegar.

- Put a couple drops of peppermint oil on the back and sides of the neck, inside of wrists, and bottom of the feet. Or add 25 drops of peppermint oil in a 1 ½-quart water bottle and use as a spray.

LIFESAVERS

- For high fevers with a severe headache and excruciating neck pain on bending the head forward, seek out immediate professional medical care to rule out meningitis.

TRIPSAVERS

- If you do develop a fever, rest and use immune support at the outset, and use the natural tips to break it as quickly as possible so as not to lose travel days unnecessarily.

FLU (See Also Colds, Cough and Bronchitis, Sore Throat)

These viral bugs can really bring you to your knees when you're traveling. They can be remarkable tenacious and virulent, lasting up to weeks. Often we find that homeopathy wipes out flu symptoms overnight.

HOMEOPATHY

- ***Bryonia alba*** (Hops): Dry, chapped, parched mouth and lips. Great thirst for cold drinks. Hard, dry cough. All symptoms worse from any movement. Joint, muscle ache, headache. Rib pain from coughing.

Grumpy. Wants to go home.

- *Eupatorium perfoliatum* (Boneset): Deep aching, soreness, and bruising in the bones as if they were broken. Muscle aches. Eyeballs feel sore.

- *Ferrum phosphoricum* (Iron phosphate): The very first stage of the flu, (without clear symptoms). High fever with flushed face and red cheeks or pale face.

- **Gelsemium** (Yellow jasmine): Dizzy, drowsy, droopy, and dull. Exhausting flu. Muscle aches throughout body. Mind dull. Eyelids heavy. Blurred vision. Just want to lie down and sleep. Chills up spine. Little thirst. Sore throat.

- **Oscillococcinum** *(Duck heart and liver)*: The first sign of the flu when specific symptoms have not yet appeared. It is available only in 200C potency, so usually only one dose is needed. If you do relapse, take another dose. No need to take all six tubes in the package in order to get relief. Save the rest for the next flu.

- *Rhus tox.* (Poison ivy): Flu with extreme muscle aching and stiffness. Desire to stretch, move around. Flu from overexertion or getting cold and wet.

🚫 **PREVENTION**

- We recommend to all of our patients an up-to-date *Influenzinum* once each fall to prevent the flu for the year. Or take *Oscillococcinum* at the first sign of the flu.

- Immune support, such as echinacea, elderberry, Osha root, Reishi and other mushrooms. We recommend Immune-a-Day and Olive Leaf Relief to our patients. Start taking at the very first sign of flu and continue every two hours for a few days, or until the symptoms pass. www.healthyhomeopathy.com/shop

- A neti pot to irrigate the sinuses can be helpful to prevent upper respiratory flu.

- If your travel partner has the flu, do not share utensils, dishes, eyeglasses. Cover the mouth when sneezing and dispose of used tissues.

MORE NATURAL TIPS

- You can still begin immune support once you get the flu—just hit it hard.
- Plenty of fluids, especially hot ginger tea or hot lemon juice with honey.
- Avoid sweets while you have a cold or flu—they weaken your immunity.
- Vitamin A 25,000 IU, Vitamin E 400 IU, and zinc 30-50 mg can help.
- Or gargle with ¼ c. apple cider vinegar , ½ c. warm water and 1 tsp. honey.
- Saunas and steam baths, steamy showers, vaporizers can help.
- Zinc lozenges.

LIFESAVERS

- Thousands of people do die from the flu each year, internationally, but they are mostly already ill or highly susceptible. We are not proponents of flu vaccines, partly because of their mercury preservative, thimerosal, and because homeopathy is so effective for the flu. Do take sensible precautions if you are elderly, weak, or immune-compromised, and decide for yourself. Be aware of serious international flu epidemics.

TRIPSAVERS

- We cannot begin to count how many times natural immune support capsules have kept us healthy while others around us were dropping like flies with bad colds and flu!

FOOD POISONING

If you get an attack of nausea with profuse vomiting soon after eating, it is likely due to food poisoning. You may also experience appetite loss, abdominal cramping, diarrhea, sweating, and fever. Not fun!

The more you mix and mingle with the locals, the more you may consume some off-the-beaten track dish that messes with your digestion. It can be viewed as bad manners to refuse what is considered to be a local delicacy. A close buddy, while traveling through the Andes, was invited by an indigenous Peruvian family to share in a delicacy: *cuy* (guinea pig). Being a vegetarian for years, he gazed down, horrified, at the poor, little creature staring up at him from the plate, with

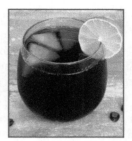
Chicha morada

eyes, paws, and nails intact. He was speechless, but his mountain-guide girlfriend nudged him under the table, making it clear that he *must* partake, or else his behavior would be worse than rude. It was a good thing he had already proven his amiability by chugging down his fair share of *chicha morada* (purple corn and pineapple beverage). Yes, he did actually eat the cuy, as custom demanded, and survived to tell us about it decades later!

Bob: We were invited to join a *campesino* family of weavers for a chicken soup lunch outside of Oaxaca, Mexico. Several hours afterwards, I was flat out with exhausting diarrhea and painful abdominal cramps. Shortly after taking a dose of *Gelsemium,* I was fine.

HOMEOPATHY

- *Agaricus* (Fly agaric): Mushroom poisoning. Twitching, jerking, or convulsions. Burning, itching, and icy coldness of extremities like frostbite.

- ***Arsenicum album*** (Arsenic): Nausea and vomiting after eating or drinking. Severe abdominal cramping. Burning pains in abdomen and rectum. Tremendous anxiety, restlessness, fear of death. Chilly. Wants sips of water.

- *Botulinum*: Food poisoning from canned food. Cramping pain in stomach. Difficulty swallowing and breathing. Weakness, staggering gait, dizziness, slurred speech. Weakness of facial muscles. Choking sensation. Paralysis.

- *Gelsemium* (Yellow jasmine): Dizzy, drowsy, droopy, and dull after ingesting old or bad food.

- **Ipecac.** (Ipecac root): Constant nausea. Violent vomiting. Sinking sensation in stomach and nausea at the smell of food. Abdominal cramping. Clear tongue.

- *Nux vomica* (Quaker buttons): Sick after eating too much rich food or drinking too much alcohol. Heartburn, burping, nausea, unproductive vomiting. Constipation without any urge for a bowel movement. Chilly, Irritable, impatient.

- **Podophyllum** (May apple): Abdominal cramping with rumbling, explosive diarrhea, exhaustion. Yellowish-green diarrhea shoots all over toilet. Worse 5AM. Rumbling, gurgling before stool. Liver pain. Worse sour fruit, food, drink.

- **Pulsatilla** (Windflower): Indigestion from eating rich or fatty foods, ice cream, pork. Heaviness in abdomen. Bloating, belching, gas. No thirst. Likes rich foods, ice cream. Clingy, weepy. Worse in warm, stuffy rooms. Better from fresh air.

- *Pyrogen* (Decomposed beef): Food poisoning from rotten meat. Septic state with fever and bad-smelling discharges. Bloating, cramping, black diarrhea.

- *Urtica urens* (Stinging nettle): Food poisoning or allergic reaction from shellfish. Intense itchy, stinging, burning hives worse from bathing and warmth.

- **Veratrum album** (White hellebore): Violent abdominal cramping with vomiting and profuse, painful, forceful watery diarrhea. Diarrhea followed by exhaustion, cold sweat, feels icy cold. Desires ice, sour, juicy, salty.

PREVENTION

- Wash your hands and utensils with warm, soapy water or a disinfectant gel, if you do not have access to safe, running water, or you are camping.

- Use a water-purifying ultra-violet device, such as a SteriPEN, or water purification tablets of iodine (Potable Aqua) or chlorine dioxide (Aquamira) to make the water used to wash produce safe.

- Peel fruits and vegetables unless you know you can trust the water. Be particularly careful of salads.

- Check for food spoilage more carefully in tropical areas without ice and refrigeration.

F

- Don't eat wild mushrooms unless you know

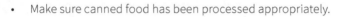

Indian buffet. Those spices can be potent!

clearly which are safe and which are poisonous.

- Make sure canned food has been processed appropriately.

- Avoid raw meat or seafood that is at all old or spoiled.

- If traveling without refrigeration, avoid mayonnaise (and other raw egg products) and toss perishables as soon as they go bad.

- Avoid eating meat if you have doubts about the hygiene of the facilities.

- Avoid eating seafood from a beach with a red tide warning.

- If you are not sure whether the local cheese is safe, better to go with hard, processed or cream cheese rather than unprocessed, soft cheese.

- When eating at a hot food buffet, go early rather than at the end of the day, when the food has been sitting in the steam tables for hours.

MORE NATURAL TIPS

- Pack lightweight protein bars to have in an emergency.

- Take a probiotic that doesn't need refrigeration or find fresh, local, live yogurt.

- If you have any question about the chicken, fish, beef, or pork that is available, play it safe and go vegetarian.

- If you are in a group food preparation situation without hot water or a dishwasher, at the very least, insist on a chlorine dish dipping station.

LIFESAVERS

- Food poisoning can be especially serious and life threatening for young children, during pregnancy, older adults, and those with compromised immune systems. We just saw a new child patient who nearly died of an *E. coli* infection.

F

TRIPSAVERS

- Moms: DO breastfeed while traveling with your infant! It is widely accepted throughout the world, essential to keep your baby healthy, and prevents disease! A sick baby can spoil your trip and introducing cow's milk too early can set the stage for ear infections, allergies, asthma, and eczema.

FRACTURES

If you break a bone, do not move or manipulate it unnecessarily. Get an X-ray. Above all, make sure it is properly casted or splinted by a medical professional. A sloppy job can leave you with a deformity and pain for life.

HOMEOPATHY

- *Arnica* (Leopard's bane): Use FIRST for any trauma. Bleeding, painful injury. Sore, bruised feeling in the muscles as if beaten. Bluish-black bruise under the skin. Compound fractures that bleed. The injured person refuses help.

- **Calcarea phosphorica** (Calcium phosphate): Fractures that do not heal well after a long time. Non-union of broken bones. Bones are soft, thin, brittle.

- *Eupatorium perfoliatum* (Boneset): Deep aching in the bones. Sore and bruised feeling in the muscles. Restless but keeps still because it hurts to move.

- **Symphytum** (Knitbone): The BEST medicine to use for fractures. Use after the bones are set properly. Produces rapid bone healing.

PREVENTION

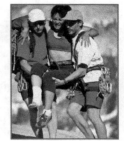

- If you have problems with balance, or have osteoporosis, take extra precautions to avoid falls.

- When hiking, wear good boots and use 1 or 2 walking sticks. Take good gear, choose trails well, know weather conditions, and be aware of your limits.

- During your travels, and for life, take a high potency, comprehensive multivitamin with minerals.

- Your serum Vitamin D level should be at least 40, preferably 60. This is easy to check by a blood test, and to correct, by supplementing with 2,000-5,000 IU/day.

MORE NATURAL TIPS

- Increase your protein intake to promote post-fracture healing. Eat well. Avoid pop, which can leach calcium out of your bones.

- Avoid aspirin and ibuprofen! Non-steroidal anti-inflammatory drugs including these, interfere with inflammatory prostaglandins, which are needed for initial tissue repair and subsequent fracture healing. If you need something more for pain relief (unlikely in our experience), take Tylenol.

- Instead take natural anti-inflammatory alternatives such as bromelain (taken away from meals), curcumin (turmeric), and bioflavonoids such as quercetin.

- Vitamin C and omega-3 fatty acids reduce inflammation.

- Smoking and alcohol consumption can diminish bone health.

- Take a high-quality, comprehensive multivitamin and mineral.

- Calcium 1000mg and Magnesium 500mg/day can build strong bones.

- Vitamins C, D, and K are essential in laying down mineral in new bone.
- There may be local herbs, such as horsetail, burdock, or others that will promote healing of fractures.

 LIFESAVERS

No need to be the crazy one whose bungee cord breaks just before rebounding. Adventure is great, but don't risk your life. There can be a temptation to do things while traveling that you would never do at home (like when we went tandem parapenting off a cliff in Queenstown, New Zealand). If you are engaging in extreme sports, make sure you have a responsible, experienced guide. And good karma!

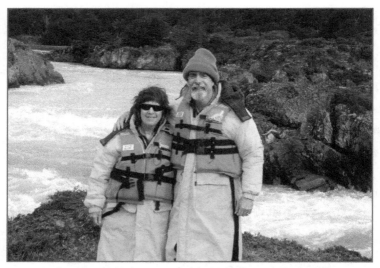

Surviving the Methow, we rafted the Lower Trancura. Pucón, Chile

Bob: We celebrated my 40th birthday with an exciting, 3-hour river rafting trip on the Methow River in Eastern Washington that could have been the end of me. We found out the hard way that the guide had never before been on the river. He led us promptly into the dreaded "black hole" whirlpool that we were warned about during the briefing. The raft turned suddenly on end, and I found myself catapulted over the side into the icy cold river. While airborne, I instinctively grabbed the rope that ran the perimeter of the boat, which keep everyone but me safely inside. Fortunately one of our fellow rafters had the presence of mind to grab hold of me and pull me back into the boat. This was in violation of the original instructions of the guides which were, in case of capsize, to push the one who was overboard straight down into the water so he would pop back up due to buoyancy, and be easier to rescue. I had a genuine, white-knuckle experience until we reached the shore. Not my favorite birthday present! (A dose of *Aconite* would have helped a lot to calm the fear and shock in these circumstances, had we brought our kit along for the ride.)

TRIPSAVERS

- If you suffer a fracture while traveling, have it taken care of immediately. Not just the bone setting but, if you will not be returning home within a month or so, get expert advice on exercise and physical therapy.

FRIGHT

Travel can be unpredictable, even with the best laid plans. Whether your wallet or gear is stolen, you are a victim of a mugging, you suffer an accident or a near miss at the hands of an irresponsible or inebriated driver, a kidnapping, terrorist attack, earthquake, volcanic eruption, or you become lost—any of these can be terrifying, and can result in PTSD (post-traumatic stress disorder). Homeopathy can be remarkably, quickly effective after such events and can often prevent future psychological trauma.

HOMEOPATHY

- **Aconite** (Monkshood): Sudden fright, fear, shock. Illness after a fright. Extreme fear of death. Tremendous restlessness. Panic. Terror-stricken. Anguished. Claustrophobia, agoraphobia, fear of crowds. Rapid heartbeat and violent heart palpitations. Shortness of breath. Flushed face. Very thirsty for cold water. First medicine to give after natural disaster, or terrorist attack.

- *Arnica* (Leopard's bane): Fright or shock after traumatic injury. Sore, bruised feeling. Fear of being touched. Refuses help. Wants to be left alone.

- *Arsenicum album* (Arsenic): Tremendous anxiety. Fear of death. Restlessness. Fears robbers. Burning pains. Insomnia after midnight. Very cold.

- *Gelsemium* (Yellow jasmine): Stage fright. Dizzy, drowsy, droopy, and dull. Muscles ache. Illnesses following fright or bad news. Diarrhea from fright.

- *Stramonium* (Thorn apple): Terrified, especially of the dark, deep water, being alone, wild animals, dogs, and ghosts. Clinging. Rage and violence if attacked or provoked.

PREVENTION

- Be careful if you are a woman traveling alone, in a dangerous country or area, out alone at night, or you seem to be pursued by someone suspicious.

- Research your destination and know what is safe to do and what is not.

- If alone, let others know where you are going and give contact information.

- Carry passport and money in a money belt, take padlocks for rooms if advised, luggage locks, and bicycle-type locks if you need to spend the night in an airport, or somewhere that you do not feel safe.

- Take care withdrawing large amounts of cash from cash machines in dark, deserted areas.

- Be aware of pickpockets in crowded markets and gatherings. Take care with cameras and other valuables.

- Check travel advisories in political hot spots and change your plans if there is significant political unrest.

- If you are working or traveling in dangerous places, register with your local embassy or consulate.

- Stay away from large or volatile political gatherings if there is conflict.

- Avoid rowdy bars or discos, especially after midnight. Inebriated patrons who aren't thinking clearly can be prey to muggers or wallet snatchers.

- Above all, follow your intuition—If you don't feel safe, leave! Or don't go. Seek help immediately if your inner voice registers alarm.

F

MORE NATURAL TIPS

- Take long, deep breaths and assure yourself that all is well.

- If alone and feel in danger, seek help immediately.

- Bach Flower Rescue Remedy can calm your nerves and your fears.

- Take sedative herbs such as passionflower, skullcap, and hops.

- Chamomile tea is calming and relaxing.

TRIPSAVERS

- In case of a crime, file a police report. **Bob:** I inadvertently dropped my wallet outside the produce market in Pucón, where we live. I looked exhaustively around the vicinity and asked the vendor, to no avail. I proceeded to the *carabineros* (police station) and filed a report, but was told it hadn't been turned in. I returned again the next day to the police station. Still no wallet had turned up. We would have normally notified our credit card provider, but Judyth had a feeling the wallet would be found. We checked online banking and no fraudulent charges had been made. The weekend passed.

The following Monday we showed up at the *Registro Civil* to report the loss of my *cedula* (Chilean I.D. card). Before approaching the local official, we spotted an acquaintance whom we had met weeks before at a workshop. He inquired as to what we were doing. there, and I responded that I was getting a new card to replace

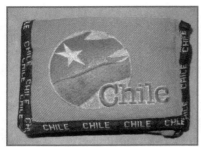

Bob's famous lost and found wallet

the one in my lost wallet. He immediately questioned me, "Is your wallet blue?" "As a matter of fact (in Spanish), yes it is." "And," he continued, "are there lots of credit cards in it?"

Now, really curious, I replied, "Yes, how did you know?" "Because I was at the *carabineros* the other day and a young woman turned it in." We hightailed it back to the police station and asked for the wallet. They told us it hadn't been turned in, but when we insisted, they led us to several drawers of found items in the back room. We opened a few drawers and there it was! They might have been incompetent, but going back to the police station did result in the resurfacing of my wallet, which was quite a relief!

FROSTBITE

When your tissues become so cold that they freeze, at temperatures below freezing for prolonged periods of time without adequate clothing, gloves, and footwear, you've got frostbite. High winds and high altitude put you more at risk, as well as poor-fitting boots. Fingers, toes, nose, and ears are most vulnerable. The affected body part becomes cold, hard, and white. It is usually not painful until it warms up again. Redness, itching, throbbing, and blistering may occur upon re-warming.

HOMEOPATHY

- **Agaricus** (Fly agaric): Burning, itching, redness, and swelling of the skin, ears, nose, and extremities. Itching of toes and feet. Skin is painful when cold. Hands and feet feel frozen.

- *Nitric acid:* Mild frostbite. Splinter-like pains. Affected areas are inflamed, itching, skin is cracked. Painful fingers and toes. Great anxiety about health.

- *Pulsatilla* (Windflower): Burning, sticking, itching pains in frozen parts. Parts are swollen, bluish red, painful. Area is hot to the touch with lack of sensation.

- *Secale* (Ergot of rye): Gangrene from frostbite.

- *Zincum* (zinc): Frostbite that feels worse from rubbing. Nose is often affected and remains red for a long time. Toes are the main area of frostbite. Very restless legs, especially at night in bed.

PREVENTION

- Bundle up in layers!

- Stay DRY. Wet skin will freeze more quickly than dry skin at the same temperature.

- Place cold hands in armpits or next to groin to warm them.

- Don't touch metal in severe cold because it can intensify frostbite.

- Take care to buy boots that dry quickly and fit well with proper socks.

- Alcohol and smoking inhibit circulation, so avoid them.

- Mittens are warmer than gloves.

- Avoid jewelry and tight clothing when in very cold weather.

- When your skin is intensely chilled, it is very vulnerable to burning. When warming up by a campfire or a heat lamp, avoid overexposure.

MORE NATURAL TIPS

- Take cayenne pepper orally to improve blood circulation, or use cayenne foot warmers in your boots.

LIFESAVERS

- Frostbite is usually treatable, but it can be fatal when accompanied by hypothermia. This occurs when your body temperature falls below 95F.

TRIPSAVERS

- If you will be evacuated promptly, thaw the area, but NEVER rub it. Reheat the affected part by immersing in water heated to 104F (40C). As the frostbitten area warms up, the pain can be intense. Remove any rings because the thawed part will swell. Keep clean and dry and cover with a dry dressing to decrease risk of infection.

GAS

Belching, passing gas (flatulence), and abdominal bloating can be painful, uncomfortable, and embarrassing.

G

HOMEOPATHY

- **Carbo vegetabilis** (Charcoal): Tremendously bloated with gas. Belching. Collapsed, weak, or exhausted with difficulty breathing. Wants to be fanned. Very cold with blueness of the lips. Worse from rich food.

- **Colocynthis** (Bitter cucumber): Agonizing, cutting gas pains alleviated by bending over double, bringing the knees to the chest, or putting pressure and warmth on the abdomen. Worse from eating, especially fruit. Easily offended.

- **Lycopodium** (Club moss): Gas and bloating worse right after a meal and worse from even a little food. Abdomen sensitive to pressure. All symptoms are worse on the right side. Pain in liver and across abdomen from right to left. Worse beans, cabbage. Desire for sweets and room-temperature drinks.

- *Nux vomica* (Quaker buttons): Unsuccessful attempts to pass gas, with straining. Muscle tension, arched back. Wakes at 3AM with gas pains. Constipated with terrible straining for BM. Chilly. Irritable, impatient.

- *Pulsatilla* (Windflower): Gas from eating ice cream, pork, fats, rich food. Bloating from gas. Worse rich foods, hot, stuffy rooms. No thirst. Moody.

PREVENTION

- Lactaid and Beano products can relieve gas from intolerance to the lactose in dairy products or beans.

- Eliminate gas-forming foods from the diet, such as beans, potatoes, sweets, and carbonated drinks.

- Try steaming, baking, or stir frying veggies rather than eating them in salads.

- Try following the principles of food combining if you are gas-prone: Avoid combining proteins and carbs at the same meal. Eat fruit by itself, not as a dessert. For melons: "Eat them alone or leave them alone."

- Eat slowly. Do not watch T.V. or read the news while eating.

MORE NATURAL TIPS

- Charcoal absorbs gas. Charcoal capsules (two every four hours) or, in a pinch, burnt toast, can often take the edge off the discomfort.

- Lying on your back while bringing your knees to the chest is a 5000+ - year-old yoga position known to yogis as the "Wind-relieving pose." Be prepared. It works!

- Massaging the abdomen in a clockwise direction helps pass gas.

- Babies may be burped over the shoulder.

- If constipation is treated, gas often resolves.

- Triphala, an Ayurvedic combination of three fruits, is an excellent digestive aid.

- Psyllium husk (Isabgol in India) can help relieve gas. Drinks LOTS of water while taking it.

- Fresh, live, local yogurt, or a probiotic in capsule form, replenishes normal gut flora. It is essential after taking antibiotics for digestive complaints.

- Other widely available kitchen spices to use for gas: ginger, either the fresh root or as a tea; caraway, fenugreek, garlic, and parsley.

- Colonic irrigation, now and then, can improve digestion and relieve gas.

LIFESAVERS

- More serious abdominal problems are sometimes mistaken for simple gas pains. If gas does not resolve within six to twelve hours, or is very severe, or accompanied by fever, nausea, and vomiting, get medical attention.

TRIPSAVERS

- At higher altitudes, the barometric pressure is lower and trapped gases expand, causing bloating, then lots of passing of gas. If you are in close quarters, trying to create a romantic ambience, or are a self-conscious person, keep your gas-prevention supplies (homeopathic kit, charcoal, etc.) close at hand to avoid embarrassment of the loss of a travel love affair.

GRIEF

You never know when you will experience death, illness, or trauma of a loved one, a relationship breakup, or a catastrophic event while traveling. It can be devastating to be alone and far from home at such a time. Homeopathy can be invaluable. Some good friends, who are also homeopaths, happened to arrive for their long-awaited trip to Bali, just at the time of the terrorist attack during which a number of Australian and other tourists were killed. Instead of relaxing on beaches and visiting exotic temples, they generously devoted their time to treating the victims, their family members, and their companions.

HOMEOPATHY

- *Ignatia* (St. Ignatius bean): Uncontrollable crying, sobbing, sighing, mood swings, appetite loss, lump in throat after a grief, hurt, disappointment.

- *Natrum muriaticum* (Sodium chloride): Grief or disappointed relationship. Feelings hurt very easily. Prefers to cry alone. Desire for salt, pasta.

- *Phosphoric acid*: Exhaustion and apathy from grief, emotional shock, burnout, disappointed love. Painless diarrhea. Strong desire for cold, fizzy drinks.

 PREVENTION

- When a loved one is seriously ill or dying, it can be very hard to know whether or not to go ahead with your trip. If you know ahead that your trip may be hanging in the air, purchase a flexible airfare and trip insurance, allowing reimbursement in case of cancellation. It can be emotionally draining to travel last minute, just before a surgery or death. It is impossible to prevent the grief, but taking the right homeopathic medicine, getting sleep and good food, can really help.

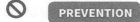 **MORE NATURAL TIPS**

- If homeopathic medicines are not available, try Rescue Remedy.

- Calming, sedative herbs such as chamomile, passionflower, skullcap, and hops can be helpful.

 LIFESAVERS

- Each moment is precious. We never know what the next moment will bring. One of our brightest homeopathic students perished in TWA flight 800, which crashed soon after takeoff from JFK into the Atlantic near East Moriches, N.Y. in July, 1996, killing all 230 people aboard.

- While traveling in Ecuador, we met an Indian IT consultant who just missed being in the Twin Towers on 9-11, thanks to a golf date with his boss.

- A brilliant, dynamic young DJ, son of our friends, just about to marry and to begin performing internationally, died instantly when his Bangkok taxi was rear-ended. His fiancé was hospitalized with a fractured sacrum. We can act wisely to try to prevent tragedy, but, in the end, everyone has his time.

- Even if you are normally a caregiver, this is the time to reach out for help. Be it the Red Cross, a Good Samaritan, a psychologist, counselor, spiritual guide, or just a shoulder to cry on, be open to receiving kindness and compassion for your loss or trauma. This is especially true if your traveling companion suffers a death or trauma. Get help!

HAY FEVER

The sneezing, runny nose, and nasal congestion of hay fever can really ruin a trip. But, with our recommendations, you don't need to be miserable.

H

HOMEOPATHY

- **Allium cepa** (Onion): Thin, watery, irritating nasal discharge that runs like a faucet. As if you were peeling an onion. Bland eye discharge.

- *Arundo* (Reed): Maddening itching of the palate and nostrils, causing sneezing.

- **Euphrasia** (Eyebright): Hay fever focuses on the eyes. Hot, irritating discharge from the eyes, bland nasal discharge. Eyes watery and sensitive to light. Frequent sneezing. Headache in forehead.

- *Natrum muriaticum* (Sodium chloride): Watery or egg-white nasal discharge. Watery eyes, swollen lids. Loss of smell and taste. Nose alternates between profuse discharge and stopped up. Cold sores. Crack in middle, lower lip.

- *Nux vomica* (Quaker buttons): Runny nose in daytime and outdoors. Dry nose at night. Violent sneezing. Sniffles. Worse being outside. Irritable, impatient.

- **Sabadilla** (Mexican grass): Attacks of violent sneezing. Watery nasal discharge worse from the smell, or even thought of, flowers. Itching and tickling in the nose with a thin, irritating discharge.

- *Sulphur* (Sulfur): Watery, burning nasal discharge when outdoors. Nose is plugged indoors. Frequent sneezing. Burning pain in the eyes.

- *Wyethia* (Poison weed): Extreme itching in the throat, palate, and nose. Terrible itching at back of sinuses. Desire to scratch palate with tongue. Back of throat is dry and burning. Throat feels swollen.

 PREVENTION

- Use an air purifier to remove pollens from the air.

- Vacuum your living and work areas more often during hay fever season.

- Wraparound sunglasses can prevent pollen from entering your eyes.

 MORE NATURAL TIPS

- Take bioflavonoids, such as quercetin, daily if exposed.

- Herbal *Urtica urens* (stinging nettles) is often helpful.

- Sip a glass of two Alka-Seltzer Gold tablets dissolved in water or drink 1t baking soda dissolved in a glass of water.

- Take 500mg buffered Vitamin C every two hours (up to 3000mg/day) until symptoms pass.

- We recommend, to our patients, herbal *Euphrasia* eye drops, a quercetin nasal spray, and an herbal antihistamine containing hesperidin.

 TRIPSAVERS

- If you are a serious hay fever sufferer, plan your trips away from pollen season at your destination. If that is not possible, and you find yourself sneezing desperately with no relief, choose an indoor activity for the day.

HEADACHE (Acute)

We are talking about acute, short-lived headaches here, rather than chronic or recurrent headaches, which require more complex, constitutional homeopathic care. If headaches are very painful, persistent, or recurrent, it may indicate a more serious underlying problem, such as a brain tumor or aneurysm.

HOMEOPATHY

- **Belladonna** (Deadly nightshade): Sudden, maddening, violent, severe, throbbing headaches worse on the right side. Extreme sensitivity to light, noise, and the least jarring. Headaches from sunstroke. Glass eyes. Fiery, red, hot, dry face. Worse 3PM. Better in a silent, dark room. Desires lemons.

- *Bryonia* (Hops): Bursting, splitting headache worse from any motion. Parched mouth and lips. Holds the head to keep it from moving. Better pressure or lying on painful side. Worse 9PM. Irritable. Wants to go home. Thirst for cold drinks.

- *Gelsemium* (Yellow jasmine): Headache after fright or stage fright. Dizzy, drowsy, droopy, and dull. Head heavy, hard to lift. Muscle aching entire body.

- **Glonoine** (Nitroglycerine): Violent bursting, throbbing, pounding headache, especially after exposure to the sun. Sunstroke. Confused, bewildered.

- *Natrum muriaticum* (Sodium chloride): Headaches after disappointment or grief. Pain in forehead. Throbbing or sensation of hammers knocking on the brain. Worse sun or heat. Feelings hurt easily. Desires salt.

- *Spigelia* (Pinkroot): Violent, burning pains affecting nerves, especially the facial nerve. Worse left side. Sensation of a hot needle, poker, or wire in or above the left eye. Extreme sensitivity to touch. Worse sun, smoke.

PREVENTION

- Avoid prolonged exposure to, or overexertion in, the sun.

- Avoid monosodium glutamate (MSG) in Chinese food and many other processed foods.

- Some people get headaches from food allergies and sensitivities, such as to wheat, corn, dairy, etc.

- Do not overdo sweets.

- Avoid hangovers.

- Drink plenty of water—dehydration can trigger headaches.

- Excessive stress can produce tension headaches. Be realistic about what you take on, and find effective techniques like yoga, deep breathing, relaxation tapes, whatever works for you.

- If you are very sensitive, try to avoid overloading yourself with bright lights, smells, or stimuli.

- Make sure your prescription for eyeglasses or contacts is up to date to avoid eyestrain.

- Get enough sleep.

- Maintain good posture. Use postural aids like the Nada Chair or the YogaBack for your car. www.nadachair.com or www.yogaback. com/The_YogaBack_for_Driving/commute.html

H

MORE NATURAL TIPS

- For throbbing, congestive headaches: put an ice pack on your head or wrap a cold, wet cloth around your head, and put your hands and feet in warm water.

- Escape to a quiet, dark place where you will not be disturbed.

- For tension headaches, take a hot bath with 1 c. Epsom salt.

- Put deep pressure on the indentations at the back of the scalp just above the neck (occipital ridge). Release when the pain subsides.

- Peppermint oil on the temples often provides relief.

- Going too long without eating can result in a hypoglycemic headache.

- Switch to decaf coffee or herb tea to avoid caffeine withdrawal.

- Evaluate and balance your hormones if an imbalance is triggering your headaches.

- Neck strain after sleeping on a hotel pillow that is too hard, or with your head bobbing on the plane while trying to sleep upright, can result in headaches. Taking a good airplane pillow can make a huge difference.

 LIFESAVERS

- If you have an unusually sudden, violent headache, uncharacteristic for you, that does not let up, seek immediate medical attention to make sure it is not an aneurysm or stroke. We know of two people who went to bed with excruciating, violent headaches and never woke up, and a third who was rushed to the hospital with an aneurysm, was hospitalized for weeks, and survived.

TRIPSAVERS

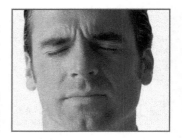

- Allow enough time at the airport for you to partake of a 15- or 30-minute chair massage, now available in many major airports.

- If the craziness of security lines and flight hassles is getting the best of you, go find a quiet seat off by itself and do deep relaxation or meditation. A number of airports have chapels, meditation rooms, or quiet areas where you can chill out and rest body, mind, and soul.

HEAD INJURY

Seek medical attention immediately for any severe head injury, especially if there is disorientation, loss of consciousness, dilated pupils, severe pain, excessive sleepiness, bleeding from the head, eyes or ears, visual disturbance, stupor, or a fracture. Afterwards, homeopathy can be extremely beneficial.

HOMEOPATHY

- ***Arnica*** (Leopard's bane): Any serious head trauma, especially with bruising. Shock. Give FIRST for any head injury. Concussion with bleeding and bruising of the tissues and brain. Black eyes. Sore, bruised feeling as if beaten. Bluish-black discoloration under skin. Worse touch. Refuses help.

- ***Helleborus*** (Black hellebore): Dullness and mental confusion after a head injury. Stupefied, bewildered. Staring into space. Not all there. Slow to answer questions, process information. Indifferent or anguished. Worse 4PM to 8PM.

- *Hypericum* (St. John's Wort): Head injury and concussion, especially if the spinal nerves are involved. Injury to spinal cord and nervous system. Shooting pains. Dizziness, headache, seizures, memory loss after head injury. Numbness and tingling.

- ***Natrum sulphuricum*** (Sodium sulfate): Second common medicine, after Arnica, for head injuries. After-effects of head injury, especially convulsions, headaches, or severe depression. Crushing pain back of head. Scalp sensitive to combing hair. Indigestion with headache.

PREVENTION

- It can be challenging to insist on safety when in an unfamiliar culture, do not speak the language, and do not know the area. If you don't feel fully comfortable in a situation, don't participate.

- Buy and use helmets or approved protective gear for baseball/ softball (when batting), cycling, football, hockey, horseback riding, powered recreational vehicles, skateboards/scooters, skiing, and wrestling.

H

- When traveling, do not engage in these activities without proper equipment.

- When considering extreme sports adventures while traveling, choose a reputable company and make sure you feel good about the guide. If not, don't go. The bungee cord that breaks, the parachute that doesn't open the aqualung without full tanks, or the guide thinking of his girlfriend instead of your safety, could be yours!

- Drive defensively.

- Do not dive into pools of any kind unless you know they are safe and at least 12 feet deep.

- When renting cars in foreign countries, know the rules of the road, purchase good insurance, drive defensively, and always use seatbelts.

- DO NOT drive when drinking. If there is no alcohol-free designated driver, walk or take a taxi or other public transportation.

- If you are in public transportation on steep, winding roads and the driving scares you, get out and find alternate transportation.

- Don't drive cars or machines if you are lightheaded or unsteady.

MORE NATURAL TIPS

- Apply an ice pack to a closed head injury to reduce swelling.

- Give clear fluids unless unconscious or vomiting.

- Treat open wounds with first aid.

- Treat for shock, if necessary. (See SHOCK, page 195)

- If you feel shaky, lightheaded, or pressure in your head, lemon balm, chamomile, skullcap, hops, and passionflower teas can relax.

LIFESAVERS

- It is easy to go with the excitement of the moment when you are traveling, especially in exotic environments and where extreme sports are the norm. Or to hop into vehicles with irresponsible, unskilled, or drunk drivers. We cannot emphasize enough: pay attention, be careful. Your life may depend on it. If you do suffer a head injury, unless you are sure you are fine, get immediate medical attention.

TRIPSAVERS

- Travel insurance can be extraordinarily helpful for medical emergencies or problems.

- AirMed evacuation can save your life if you have a serious accident outside the U.S. and need hospitalization, as well as getting you back home. www.airmed.com

HEAD LICE

H

These maddening, persistent bugs are no fun and can be very difficult to eradicate. **Judyth:** I had to deal with these buggers twice. The second time, I caught them from an airplane seat on the way back from India. You know you've got them if your head starts itching annoyingly and won't stop. A magnifying glass will reveal tiny, whitish eggs (nits) that stick to the hair follicles. You may see small, red bumps or sores on the back of the neck and scalp.

HOMEOPATHY

- We have not used homeopathy for head lice, so will stick to other approaches. We talk below about children and head lice, but the same precautions and treatments apply to adults. The conventional treatments, such as Nix or Rid, are very strong, toxic, require re-treatment, and may not be available if you are in an isolated area.

PREVENTION

- Teach your kids to avoid sharing combs, hairbrushes, hats, scarves, towels, helmets, pillows, and sleeping bags.

- Hang up coats and hats on hooks rather than tossing onto a pile.

- Clean your child's car seats, pillows, and headphones if shared.

- With reports of head lice at your child's school, or the home of a close friend or relative, go into head lice alert mode, checking your child's scalp well.

- Don't panic unnecessarily—it could just be dandruff! Is the dandruff moving? But, if it is head lice, take a deep breath and prepare yourself for an ordeal.

MORE NATURAL TIPS

- Apply real mayonnaise or olive oil (some say Vaseline, but best to avoid petroleum products) to the scalp to smother the lice. Leave on overnight, under a shower cap, and wash out the next day. Though messy and unproven, many parents report that they are effective.

- Lavender oil or tea tree oil have been said to work.

- Ulesfia (Benzyl alcohol lotion 5%) is a non-pesticide, prescription treatment used with children over 6 months. Saturate the hair with the lotion, wash off after 10 minutes. Reapply 7 days later. Unlike head lice shampoos with pesticides, is it is thought to suffocate the lice.

- *Staphysagria* (Stavesacre) is an herbal tincture from Australia used successfully for head lice. We brought it back and used it with a couple of patients. We heard neither praise nor complaints.

TRIPSAVERS

- Head lice, though they do not cause a serious problem, are highly contagious and a problem to reckon with immediately. It is one of those conditions that, when mentioned, will turn you into a pariah in no time flat. If you have the misfortune to contract them while traveling, do NOT wait until you get home to get rid of them. You will be exposing other travelers to the dreaded bugs. It is *much* easier if you are dealing with just the clothes in your pack or suitcase! In addition to treating yourself or your family, you will need to wash *all* of your clothes and bedding in hot water and dry on the hot setting, or dry clean what is needed. Do NOT rely on hand washing to deal with lice!

H

HEMORRHOIDS

Hemorrhoids are varicose veins of the rectum, internal or external. The most annoying symptoms are itching and pain due to inflammation and swelling. There might be bright-red blood around the stool or in the toilet. They are not serious, unless the bleeding is profuse.

HOMEOPATHY

- **Aesculus** (Horse chestnut): Painful, purple external hemorrhoids. The rectum feels full of small sticks. Pain is relieved when they bleed. Pain persists long after bowel movements.

- *Aloe* (Aloe socotrina): Hemorrhoids like a bunch of grapes. Filled with blood and feel congested. Lumps of mucus in stool. Stool comes out without urging and while passing gas.

- **Collinsonia** (Stone-root): Painful, bleeding hemorrhoids. Sensation of sharp sticks or sand in rectum. Hemorrhoids with heart palpitations or swelling of the face, lips. Chronic constipation alternating with diarrhea. A feeling of heaviness in the rectum.

- **Hamamelis** (Witch hazel): Swollen, purple, blood-filled hemorrhoids. Weak veins. Sore, bruised, throbbing feeling in rectum. Lots of blood. Pain can last for hours after a bowel movement. Anus sore, raw, as if full of sticks. Nosebleeds.

- *Nux vomica* (Quaker buttons): Itching, painful hemorrhoids after too much stress, rich food, drugs, alcohol, stimulants, or chronic constipation. No urge for a bowel movement. Great straining. Rectum feels constricted. Impatient. Body feels cold.

- *Sulphur* (Sulfur): Large bunches of internal and external hemorrhoids. Itching, tender, bleeding. Anus red, sore, raw, burning, and very itchy, especially at night in bed. Stool loose, burning. Hemorrhoids worse from hot baths, showers.

H

PREVENTION

- Drink lots of water and herb tea to prevent constipation, dehydration.

- Get plenty of exercise to increase circulation to the pelvic area.

- Eat a fresh, healthy organic diet with whole grains, fruits and vegetables, high fiber. Include oat, wheat, or rice bran.

- Spicy foods may aggravate hemorrhoids.

- Minimize alcohol and caffeine.

- Keep the rectum clean.

MORE NATURAL TIPS

- Homeopathic rectal suppositories, made with the medicines on our list, can be quite effective, such as Boiron Avenoc Suppositories or Ointment. Glycerine suppositories can also provide relief.

- Sitz bath: Fill a bathtub with hot water to two inches below navel. Sit with knees bent. Stay in tub five minutes. Then squat in a tub of cold water for one minute. Repeat the cycle 2-3 times.

- Bioflavonoids 1000mg/d to strengthen capillaries and prevent fragility.

- Psyllium seed or husk (drink lots of water), flaxseed or oil, and prunes or prune juice are great to prevent constipation.

- Witch hazel applied topically to hemorrhoids can shrink them.

- Drink carrot/ginger and other fresh vegetable and fruit juices.

TRIPSAVERS

- Hemorrhoids can make long bus, train, or plane trips highly uncomfortable and travel, especially in planes, has a dehydrating effect. Go out of your way to carry a water bottle, refill it frequently, and to make pit stops often. If you are prone to constipation, pack prunes and flax bars for the road.

HEPATITIS (Acute Hepatitis A)

Viral inflammation of the liver transmitted by contaminated water, stool, blood or secretions. Symptoms include weakness, nausea, vomiting, diarrhea, appetite loss, and, in some stages, jaundice (yellow skin and whites of the eyes). We have had excellent, rapid results treating our patients with acute hepatitis. The incubation period is 15-50 days, with an average of 28 days, so you may not know you have it until after your trip.

Risk factors for Hepatitis A include:

- Use of recreational, injectable drugs
- Work exposure to the Hep A virus
- Living with someone or eat food prepared by someone infected
- Being HIV positive
- Eating raw or undercooked shellfish, such as oysters or clams
- Eating undercooked food, unpeeled fruits or veggies, or drinking tap or well water in countries where Hep A is common
- Living in a community where Hep A outbreaks are common
- Sexual contact involving fecal/oral contact

HOMEOPATHY

- **Chelidonium** (Celandine): Liver tender and enlarged. Pain extends from liver backward to the lower angle of the right shoulder blade. Right-sided symptoms. Jaundice. Nausea and vomiting better from drinking hot water. Bright yellow or clay-colored stools in hard balls or diarrhea. Bitter taste in mouth. Icy fingertips.

- **China** (Peruvian bark): Liver pain under the right ribs. Liver and spleen are swollen, enlarged. Bitter belching does not provide relief. Jaundice, bloating. Tremendous sweating, worse at night. Frothy, yellow diarrhea.

- *Lycopodium* (Club moss): Pain in liver under right ribcage. Pain goes from right to left across abdomen. Lots of bloating. Worse gassy foods, tight clothing around abdomen, and after eating. Desire for warm or room temperature drinks.

- *Mercurius* (Mercury): Enlarged liver very sore to touch and pressure. Sharp pains extend from liver to spine. Scant dark, bloody urine. Greenish, slimy stools.

- *Natrum sulphuricum* (Sodium sulfate): Sharp, stitching pains in liver. Liver sore to touch. Can't tolerate tight clothing around waist. Passes gas. Jaundice and vomits bile. Diarrhea watery and yellow. Wants yogurt. Street drug history.

- *Phosphorus*: Liver large, hard, feels full. Jaundice. Craves cold or carbonated drinks, but may vomit them when they become warm in stomach.

PREVENTION

- Hepatitis A is a vaccination that we DO recommend. The vaccine is typically given in two doses—Initial and a booster 6-12 months later. It is recommended for those working or traveling in areas with high rates of infection. These include Africa, Asia (except Japan), the Mediterranean, Eastern Europe, the Middle East, Mexico, Central and South America, and parts of the Caribbean. If you are traveling to these areas sooner than a month after your first shot, a preventive dose of immunoglobulin (IG) is recommended. If you are traveling short-term to these areas, you may request the IG instead of the hepatitis vaccine.

- Do not share dishes, utensils, toothbrushes or towels.

- Peel and wash fruits and vegetables.

- Avoid raw or undercooked meat and fish.

- Ask for beverages to be served without ice.

- Either drink bottled water, where advised, or boil or safely purify tap water for drinking.

- Wash your hands often and with warm water and soap, especially after using the toilet, changing diapers, and before preparing or eating food.

- To avoid chronic hepatitis, practice safe sex and drug users should not share needles, which also is preventive for Hepatitis B and C.
- Laboratory workers should take precautions against Hepatitis A.

MORE NATURAL TIPS

- Eat a low-fat diet with lots of fruits and veggies, especially beets and beet greens.
- Vitamin C 1000mg 3 times/day
- Take liver herbs including dandelion root, and milk thistle
- Lipotropic factors, which include the amino acids cysteine, methionine, and inositol, help the liver break down fat.
- Liv-52 is an well-researched Ayurvedic herbal liver combination www.himalayahealthcare.com

LIFESAVERS

- Get tested to determine the type. Hepatitis A is acute with full and rapid recovery. Hepatitis B and C are more serious and can even, over time, become life threatening.

TRIPSAVERS

- A patient was so looking forward to a trip to Machu Picchu, followed by the Galapagos and the Ecuadorian Amazon. The first part of her trip, to the Andes, went fine. She then ended up in the hospital with a hepatitis-related liver abscess, and had to fly home without ever reaching her other long-awaited destinations. She returned home depleted, exhausted, and disappointed. We were able to help her regain her health, but

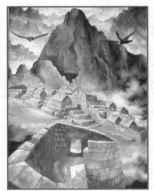

Visionary painting, Machu Picchu. Walter Huacac, Galeria de Arte Yawar Huacac

H

we wish she had contacted us from the hospital. Since we work by Skype, we can be readily available to provide information no matter where someone may be.

HIVES (See Also Allergic Reactions)

Hives are red, raised welts accompanied by itching, heat, and swelling.

HOMEOPATHY

- **Apis** (Honeybee): Hives with SWELLING, redness, stinging, and itching. Swollen, puffy face and eyelids. Large hives better from cold packs. Intolerable itching at night. Not very thirsty.

- *Rhus tox.* (Poison ivy): Hives with intense itching and burning pain. Hives from getting wet, chilled or during chills and fever. Better from heat; worse from cold, damp and overexertion. Restless.

- *Urtica urens* (Stinging nettle): Hives from shellfish with itching, burning, stinging. Prickly-heat sensation. Itchy raised, red blotches. Worse cold wet.

PREVENTION

- Avoid known triggers, to which you are susceptible, such as particular foods, plants, cosmetic and hair products, exposure to cold or to sun.

MORE NATURAL TIPS

- Self-care: Avoid scratching or rubbing. Do not break blisters. Take a cold shower and/or apply cool compresses. Wear loose, light, comfortable clothing. Keep cool by sleeping in a cool room if in a tropical climate.

- To relieve itching: Soak in warm bath with one cup of baking soda or raw oatmeal (or Aveeno).

- Sip a glass of water with 1-2 Alka-Seltzer Gold tablets dissolved or drink one t. baking soda in a glass of water. These alkalinize the body.

- Take 500mg buffered Vitamin C every two hours, up to 3g/day, until symptoms pass.

- Hesperidin supplements, such as Thorne HMC Hesperidin , contain herbal histamine-like substances. www.healthyhomeopathy.com/shop

- If other homeopathic medicines don't work, try homeopathic *Histaminum*.

 LIFESAVERS

- Serious hives can turn into life-threatening anaphylaxis within 15 minutes of the exposure to an allergen. The symptoms are intense itching and swelling, difficulty breathing due to constriction of the airways, and itching in the armpits and groin, progressing into anaphylactic shock, then death. It is a medical emergency treated with epinephrine.

 TRIPSAVERS

- If you have a history of severe allergic reactions or anaphylaxis, always carry an EpiPen (epinephrine) with you when you travel.

HYPOTHERMIA

By definition, hypothermia is when your rectal temperature falls below 95F (35C). It is not necessary to be in weather of extremely low temperature in order to become hypothermic. In fact, any temperature less than your body temperature (98.6F) could potentially be compatible with hypothermia. Wind, wet, and cold are all key players.

Risk factors:

- Cold temperatures
- Being thin with less body fat
- Fatigue, exhaustion

- Dehydration
- Being wet
- Inadequate food intake
- Inadequate clothing or equipment
- Wind
- Alcohol
- Children
- The elderly

Symptoms: Rick Curtis of the Princeton Outdoor Programs discusses the four "umbles" that indicate changes in motor coordination and levels of consciousness: stumbles, mumbles, fumbles, and grumbles. Mild hypothermia: shivering, inability to perform complex motor functions like skiing, and vasoconstriction to the periphery. Moderate: dazed, slurred speech, violent shivering, irrational behavior, apathy. Severe: shivering in periodic waves, falling to the ground due to inability to walk, curling up in a fetal position, muscle rigidity, pale skin, dilated pupils, slow pulse, death-like appearance. www.princeton.edu/~oa/safety/hypocold.shtml

HOMEOPATHY

- *Arsenicum album* (Arsenic): Extreme chilliness. Very anxious, restless, fear of death and of being alone. Desire to sip water constantly.

- *Camphora* (Camphor): Great coldness. Blue with cold. Feeling of coldness in extremities and all body parts, even tongue.

- **Carbo vegetabilis** (Charcoal): Icy coldness of the whole body, especially nose, hands, feet, knees. Cold skin, cold breath. Pale. Lips and skin bluish. Exhaustion. Wants to be fanned.

- *Secale* (Ergot of rye): Icy cold. Shivering. Blueness of gangrenous parts.

PREVENTION

- Check in with yourself and your travel companions frequently about how you are feeling if you are in a situation where hypothermia is possible.

- Add layers of dry clothing.

- Move around.

- Find protected shelter.

- Go near a fire or other external heat source

- Eat carbs for quick energy (along with proteins and fats).

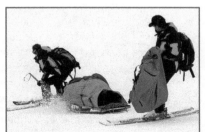

- Push fluids, especially hot liquids like warm sugar water.

- Avoid alcohol, caffeine, and smoking

- Do urinate so the body doesn't need to warm the urine in the bladder.

- Body to body contact, such as getting in a sleeping bag with dry clothing next to a person of normal body temperature who is lightly dressed.

- Wrap in multiple sleeping bags, wool blankets and clothing, Thermarest or Ensolite ground pads, and space blankets covered in plastic.

MORE NATURAL TIPS

- Cayenne foot or hand warmers or cayenne capsules can keep you warm, at least temporarily.

LIFESAVERS

- Spot Satellite or other GPS: A couple of years ago a European couple nearly died on the mountain near our Chilean home, when a bitterly cold, unexpected windstorm blew in. How did they survive?

H

157

By having a Spot Satellite emergency device and pushing the panic button, which called their Texas headquarters. A rescue was performed and their lives were spared. www.findmespot.com

- When hiking, boating, or engaging in other outdoor sports, prepare for weather changes and take layers just in case. You never know what the sky and wind will bring! Some good friends on our island went out sailing on a catamaran one beautiful day. Though they were quite experienced, the wind came up, preventing them from navigating properly, and the sun went down. They were dressed in shorts and T-shirts. Had someone not seen them and called the Coast Guard Rescue, they would not have survived.

- If the weather takes a sudden, drastic change for the worse, stay where you are and wait it out, rather than putting your life in danger. **Judyth:** One sunny morning, my ex-husband, a seasoned hiker, set off on a day hike. Heavy fog set in. Tragically, he stepped off a cliff, broke his neck, and died.

TRIPSAVERS

- Make a pact with your travel buddies to keep checking with each other as to coldness status. Once you fall into a hypothermic state, you can no longer think clearly, so prevention is literally a matter of life and death.

- Stuff a couple of clean garbage bags into your pack to use inside your pack to keep sleeping gear or clothing dry, to use, in a pinch, as a pack cover, or to cut up and pack inside wet hiking boots. **Judyth:** This trick saved me from potential hypothermia in brisk wind/driving rain conditions while backpacking in Patagonia.

INDIGESTION

Gas, belching, stomach pain, and heartburn are the common symptoms.

HOMEOPATHY

- **Arsenicum album** (Arsenic): Severe burning pains in stomach and esophagus better by drinking milk and worse after eating and drinking, especially fruit and cold food or drinks. Stomach pain at 2AM. Very anxious, restless, fear of dying. Chilly. Thirsty for sips of cold water.

- **Carbo vegetabilis** (Charcoal): Great bloating, and belching. Fainting from indigestion, passing gas. Collapsed, weak, exhausted, hard to breathe. Very cold, bluish skin. Wants to be fanned. Worse rich food.

- **Lycopodium** (Club moss): Gas, belching, bloating. Abdomen sensitive to pressure. Worse from gas-producing foods like beans, onions, cabbage. Full quickly after small amounts of food. Worse 4-8PM. Worse tight clothing around abdomen, before performing. Better warm drinks.

- **Nux vomica** (Quaker buttons): Heartburn after fats and sour food. Constipation with terrible straining. Wakes at 3AM with indigestion. Likes fat, spicy, and rich foods and stimulants. Irritable, impatient.

- **Pulsatilla** (Windflower): Heartburn and indigestion after fats, rich foods, pork, ice cream. Bloating. Stomach aches in children. Likes creamy, rich foods, peanut butter. Clingy. Worse hot, stuffy rooms.

- Sulphur (Sulfur): Heartburn after overeating or drinking. Sudden, explosive diarrhea worse at 5AM. Burning pain in stomach and esophagus. Belching with bad taste in mouth. Loose, burning stool. Smelly diarrhea (like rotten eggs), gas, sweat, and discharges. Wants sweets, fat.

PREVENTION

- Eat small meals.

- Stay with bland food at first, then work your way up the burn-your-mouth stars according to your comfort level.

- Eat lightly after 7PM.

- Cut out gas-producing foods, such as beans, potatoes, sweets, and carbonated beverages.

- Moderate your alcohol and caffeine intake.

- Smoking aggravates indigestion.

- Elevate the head of the bed 6" if you are prone to heartburn.

- If you begin to feel any symptoms, cut the spicy, fatty food and street vendor greasy fare and stick with bread, yogurt, bananas, and rice for a few days.

MORE NATURAL TIPS

- D-limonene is an effective natural citrus supplement for heartburn.

- Charcoal capsules, or burnt toast, relieve gas—2 caps every 4 hours.

- Lie on your back and bring knees to your chest (wind-relieving pose).

- Peppermint tea relieves indigestion.

- Some people use apple cider vinegar or alkaline diets for heartburn.

LIFESAVERS

- If you develop severe pain in the middle of your abdomen that comes and goes, nausea and appetite loss, a mild fever, your right lower abdomen is tender to pressure, and you still have your appendix, see a doctor to rule out appendicitis. If not treated, it can turn into peritonitis, which is life threatening.

TRIPSAVERS

- Changes in your normal diet, stress, and spicy food are all common to travel, and are triggers of indigestion and heartburn. Watch your diet from the time you leave, take any digestive aids that might be needed, and begin to introduce local, exotic, and spicy foods gradually.

- For severe pain, make sure it's not a kidney stone or kidney infection.

INSECT BITES AND STINGS

Characteristics are redness, swelling, itching, and burning or stinging pain after the bite. Remove the stinger with a flicking motion, using a fingernail or sterilized needle. Pulling it straight out may release additional poison.

Judyth: I am, unfortunately, a biting-insect magnet. Before I knew about homeopathy, I stepped on a yellow jacket's nest while walking in the woods. My ankle swelled to the size of a tennis ball. I had plans to go on a hike in the mountains the next day, and I don't give up easily. I wrapped my ankle overnight in a baking soda paste compress. The swelling was nearly gone by morning and, yes, I hiked as planned. Now I would know to take *Apis*!

HOMEOPATHY

- *Androctonus* (Scorpion): First choice for scorpion bites. If not, Ledum.

- ***Apis*** (Honeybee): Bee or other stings with SWELLING, heat, redness, and stinging. Site of sting is hot, worse from heat, and better from cold applications. Hives after a bite or sting. Itching bad at night. No thirst.

- *Caladium* (American arum): Mosquito, flea, and fly bites that burn and itch intensely.

- ***Carbolic acid:*** Anaphylactic reaction and collapse following a bee or wasp sting. Hives all over the body. Swelling of face and tongue from bee stings. Ears and throat swell shut and make breathing difficult. Water-filled blisters that burn and itch. Pale, collapsed, cold sweat. NOTE: This is a very unusual medicine not found in kits. If you know that you are prone to anaphylaxis, order ahead from a homeopathic pharmacy.

- **Formica rufa** (Red ant): Red ant bites. Joints become red, hot, and terribly painful, worse from the slightest movement. Pain migrates from one joint to another.

- **Ledum** (Marsh tea): Insect bites or stings of any kind without significant swelling, including mosquito, flea, or tick bites. Affected area is cold to touch and better from cold applications or bathing. *Ledum* may help prevent Lyme disease, so it is worth taking when first bitten by a deer tick.

- *Psorinum* (Scabies): For scabies if *Sulphur* is not effective.

- *Sulphur* (Sulfur): Specific for scabies.

- *Vespa* (Wasp): Stinging, burning pains as if pierced by red-hot needles. Redness, swelling. No recollection of having been bitten. Seizures after wasp stings with loss of consciousness and staring into space.

PREVENTION

- Once you get a bee sting, you can prevent the venom from becoming more toxic by scraping the stinger off immediately with a credit card or other firm-edged object, rather than removing with tweezers.

- Make yourself less palatable to those darned mosquitoes: Wash with soap followed by using deodorant (mosquitoes are attracted by strong body odors). Breathe (mosquitoes are attracted to carbon dioxide). Not much you can do about this one! Don't move. Mosquitoes go after a moving target. Don't sweat (they love those hot, sticky climates). Good luck!

- Wear white or khaki clothing (research shows that they are most drawn to dark colors, especially blue). Go fragrance-free (Bees supposedly love floral scents.) Avoid skin-care products containing alpha hydroxy acids (they contain the most lactic acid, which is said to be popular among the mosquito crowd). Change clothing

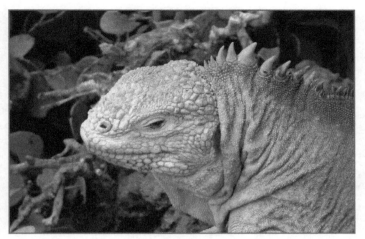

Bugs don't bug me!

and socks (they say it's the human foot bacteria that is heaven for those bugs.)

- We are wary of strong DEET-containing insect repellants. Use either herbal repellants with citronella or soybean oil or others with less than 10% DEET. We prefer the Sawyer's brand. Wash off as soon as possible. Repellants are not effective against most stinging insects like wasps, bees, and fire ants.

- Check out the Environmental Working Group's (EWG) Guide to Bug Repellants for the latest news on what is safest. www.ewg.org

- If in an area with lots of mosquitoes and biting insects for a prolonged time, spray permethrin on your outer clothing and use repellants only for exposed areas like face and hands. It lasts for 20 or so washes.

- Bug hats with netting. When we visited The Olgas, a rock formation near Ayers Rock (Uluru) in Australia, we came prepared, as the travel guides advised, with bug hats (a baseball cap with a screen that drops down to cover the face, head, and neck). There were hundreds of black flies around each of our heads, but, thankfully, they couldn't get in.

- Tuck in mosquito bed netting well around the sides of the bed.

- If in tick country, especially when camping or hiking, check your and your child's body daily for ticks and tick-caused lesions.

- Avoid anthills when setting up tents and campsites.

- If one family member contracts scabies, treat everyone else as well. Wash all bedding and clothing for a week. Some recommend applying topically a cup of kerosene/paraffin mixed with a cup of vegetable oil twice a day. Neem oil is a more natural and less toxic alternative.

 MORE NATURAL TIPS

- Apply an ice or cold, moist pack to reduce swelling and spread of poison.

- Cleanse the area with soap and water.

- *Calendula* (marigold) cream or tincture can ease itching and irritation.

- Apply a baking soda paste to the area to reduce swelling.

- In a pinch, put a dab of toothpaste on the bite to relieve swelling.

- An oatmeal bath or herbal combination of *Grindelia* and *Sarsaparilla* can relieve itching.

- *Hesperidin* supplements contain natural antihistamine.

 PREVENTION

- If you have difficulty breathing, severe swelling, or itching in the armpits and groin after an insect or spider bite, use an EpiPen or see a doctor immediately for an anaphylactic reaction. You will be given epinephrine.

 TRIPSAVERS

- If you are bitten by a tick or simply notice a red circle resembling a target around the site of a deer tick bite, seek out care immediately for Lyme Disease. **Bob:** Years ago we were jogging in rural Philadelphia, near the home of my parents, an area known for Lyme ticks.

The following day, while visiting Judyth's parents in St. Louis, I noticed the classic target lesion. We did some research at the Washington University medical school library (this was before the days of the internet), and I immediately began a course of Doxycycline, prescribed by my childhood pediatrician, who was still in practice. It is a strong antibiotic, and I was wiped out for a couple of weeks. It happened to be at the same time that we got a golden retriever puppy, and the combination of the two just about did me in. But, I never had another problem from the Lyme. As added prevention, take *Ledum* 30C at first sign of the bite and through the first two weeks. I did both.

- If at risk of a scorpion bite , take *Androctonus* (Scorpion), which can be ordered in advance from a homeopathic pharmacy.

INSOMNIA

The combination of red-eye flights, jet lag, sleeping in strange, noisy surroundings, uncomfortable beds and pillows, the snoring of seatmates, and the disorientation of leaving and arriving at airports in the middle of the night or morning, can all disrupt sleep.

HOMEOPATHY

- *Aconite* (Monkshood): Insomnia due to fright or shock. Violent heart palpitations, rapid pulse, profuse perspiration. Anxious, restless, fears death.

- **Arsenicum album** (Arsenic): Insomnia due to worry and anxiety, especially about health or money. Worse midnight to 2AM. Burning pains, chilly, restless.

- *Chamomilla* (Chamomile): Insomnia from pain, including teething. Extreme sensitivity to pain. Child is contrary, inconsolable, wants to be carried, rocked.

- **Coffea** (Unroasted coffee): Insomnia from overstimulation, excitement. Hypersensitive to emotions, pain, noise, light, touch. Wide awake at 3AM with mind full of thoughts. Mind overactive. Overemotional. Restless.

- *Gelsemium* (Yellow jasmine): Insomnia after fright or stage fright. Dizzy, drowsy, droopy, and dull. Wants to lie down to go to sleep but can't.

- *Ignatia* (St. Ignatius bean): Insomnia after grief. Uncontrollable crying, sadness, mood swings. Sobbing, sighing, lump in throat. Numbness.

- *Nux vomica* (Quaker's button): Waking at 3 AM thinking of business. Sleep loss due to heightened sensitivity to light, noise, sound or other stimuli or after too much alcohol or rich, spicy food. Irritable, impatient, chilly.

 PREVENTION

- Avoid caffeine, pop and sugar late at night.

- Take an hour of quiet or relaxation time without noise or entertainment before going to sleep. Avoid horror or action movies on the plane during the night if they tend to affect you emotionally or are too stimulating.

- A vigorous exercise program and healthy diet lead to better sleep.

- Avoid large meals after 7PM, especially very spicy, sugary, or fatty.

- Some folks say a high carbohydrate, whole-grain snack can make you fall asleep in half the time.

- On your trip, try to establish a routine bedtime and stick to it.

- Restrict overstimulating activities like T.V., computer use and gaming, and work for at least half an hour before going to bed.

- Try to get at least seven hours of quality sleep a night.

 MORE NATURAL TIPS

- Take melatonin 3 mg at bedtime.

- Drink a cup of warm milk. Eat a banana or a slice of turkey at bedtime. They all contain tryptophan, an amino acid that induces serotonin production, which induces sleep.

- Valerian, chamomile, passionflower, hops, or skullcap tea—singly, or in combination, as a tea or tincture, before bed for a sedative effect.

- Dab lavender oil on your temples before hitting the sack. Or put 5-10 drops in your bath water, if your travel accommodations have a tub.

- Deep breathing through the left nostril or alternate nostril breathing are quite effective and can be done anytime anywhere. Do for 3-10 minutes.

- Lie on the right side with your arm outstretched to induce sleep faster.

TRIPSAVERS

- Be proactive regarding sleep on international flights. Bring a travel pillow, earplugs, eyeshades, socks or booties. Wear loose, comfortable clothing. Check online for seat availability and switch to one you like better. We like exit rows, if you get to the reservation desk early enough to request one, and you are physically able, but be advised that they often have fixed armrests. We are told that Tuesdays and Wednesdays attract fewer flyers. Pick airlines that are safe, but not as popular and crowded.

- On undersold flights in non-peak season, you may be able to score three seats across in the middle section if the plane isn't crowded, so you can stretch out to sleep. Don't be afraid to trade one good seat for three, but beware of getting stuck in the middle of the plane with passengers on each side. Ask before boarding how crowded the plane is, and act accordingly.

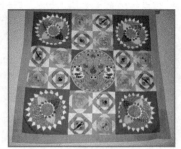

- We try to intersperse red eyes and all-night bus trips with welcoming, comfy hotels or hostels with great beds.

- Choose hotel rooms with conditions conducive to good sleep: location off the street away from

Wall art. Buena Vida Social Club B & B. El Bolson, Argentina.

noise, good pillow, mattress, and dark window shades. Some travel accommodation sites, such as TripAdvisor, encourage reviewers to indicate plum rooms. www.tripadvisor.com

JET LAG AND AIR TRAVEL STRESS

Air travel has become infinitely more grueling since 9-11. Excessively long airport security lines; the indignity of having to remove shoes, sweaters, and practically everything except underwear; whole body X-ray scans, and being patted down in your private areas if you refuse the scan; dumping your water bottle, and having to toss in the bin the trusty pocket knife that you forgot to remove from that corner of your pack. Add in the chaos of separating laptops, miniscule toiletries, and visible money belts into countless bins. Long-distance travel can exhaust the body and fray the nerves. Not to mention the discomfort of being crammed into seemingly ever more compact seats and rows.

Common symptoms are fatigue, difficult sleeping, headache, irritability, appetite loss, and constipation or diarrhea. Jet leg tends to be worse the more time zones you cross, and when traveling from west to east. Risks of air travel, especially transcontinental or transoceanic, include catching respiratory illnesses due to poor air quality on overnight red-eyes.

The most serious risk is DVT (deep-vein thrombosis—a blood clot that travels from the deep veins of the leg to the lung, causing a pulmonary embolus). Symptoms include leg pain and swelling, usually in the calf. Risk factors include pregnancy, age over 60, smoking, obesity, varicose veins, previous history of DVT or pulmonary embolus, and recent surgery or injury.

HOMEOPATHY

- *Arnica* (Leopard's bane): Sore, bruised muscles. As if you were beaten.

- *Bellis perennis* (English daisy): Bruising of the tailbone from sitting too long on long-haul airplanes where it is hard to get up and move around.

- **Cocculus** (Indian cockle): Worn out and spacey after loss of sleep or from taking care of someone. Nausea at the sight or smell of food. Weak legs.
- **Gelsemium** (Yellow jasmine): Dizzy, drowsy, droopy, dull, wiped out. Little thirst.
- *Nux vomica* (Quaker buttons): Constipation, muscle cramps. Chilly. Finally falls asleep, then wakes up miserable. Air rage. Craving for coffee and alcohol.

 PREVENTION

- Getting a good night's pre-trip sleep should get you off to a better start. Pack a couple of days before so you're not running around stuffing things into your suitcase in the wee hours of the morning before you leave.

- If you use budget travel search engines (See Travel Smart, page 29), pay close attention to the total number of hours of the trip and the number of stops. Saving a hundred dollars may not be worth the extra hassle and stress of spending hours in an airport between connections.

- Now that airlines require arrival at the airport two hours before your flight, you may just have time for a chair body massage or foot massage.

- Pack a comfy travel pillow, booties, eyeshade, and earplugs to zone out despite the screaming baby in the row behind you.

- Be savvy about seat choice. Early check-in may score you an exit-row seat. Know your plane; which seats, if any, are not reclining, and which location best meets your personal needs. Avoid seats near the lavatories, as lines often form there. Know which days of the week have the lowest fares as well as the least crowded flights.

- Few airlines offer palatable, satisfying meals anymore, unless you are a first-class or business travel passenger. You may have to fork out big bucks for a little sandwich. We take our favorite, healthy snacks from home, including trail mix, fresh fruit, and cheese. Nutritious salads, sandwiches or wraps (sodium nitrite-free), freshly squeezed juices, and smoothies are also becoming increasingly available in airports around the world. Based on your ticket class or frequent flyer status, you may be entitled to free entry into an airline board room, which may provide healthy snacks, a quiet and peaceful space for laptop use, and even a shower. We have a favorite food ritual that eases our two-day flight from Chile to Seattle, three dogs in tow. One of us claims the luggage and the dogs while the other waits in line to buy our favorite huge, shrimp, ginger, wasabi salad from Anthony's carry out. Knowing we are coming back to food we love somehow makes it all better.

- Be aware of immigration requirements, which may prevent you from entering with animal, vegetable, and dairy products.

- We take our vitamins, immune support, and homeopathic medicine kit, even for short trips, and protein powder and green drink for longer ones, if we will have access to a blender.

- It can be far more comfortable and less stressful to board early, so that you find overhead space just above you, rather than having to scramble upon arrival to collect bags stored five rows behind you.

- Airplane yoga and stretching exercises as well as walking up and down the aisles can reduce stiffness and discomfort and prevent DVT. Try a nifty airplane yoga app for your iPhone, iPod, and iPad. https://itunes.apple.com/us/app/airplane-yoga/id469614252?mt=8

- Avoiding alcohol helps reduce jet lag.

- Wet wipes take up little space and can make you feel human again on long plane trips.

- Many hotels will be happy to offer an airport pickup, especially if you are arriving in an unknown city or country or in the middle of the night.

- If possible, give yourself some down time before revving into action.

MORE NATURAL TIPS

- Set your watch to the time zone of your destination while still on

the plane. Upon arrival at your destination, take a quick nap, if necessary,
then synch yourself with the local time
as quickly as possible.

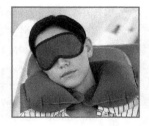

- Meditation rooms or chapels at airports
help to regain peace of mind.

- Drink plenty of non-alcoholic fluids on
the plane.

- Melatonin 3-5mg. If flying east, take in the early evening starting
a few days before your trip, then a bit later at the local bedtime
until you get adjusted to the new time zone. If flying west, take at
bedtime once you land until you are in synch with the schedule of
your destination.

- Light therapy: If traveling east, across up to six time zones: Get out
in bright sunlight during the morning the first few days after arrival,
or artificial light if there is no sun. If traveling west, up to six time
zones: Exposure to bright light at the end of each day. If crossing
over six time zones in either direction: Avoid bright light until the
middle of the day.

- Sleep herbs, including passionflower, valerian, and hops, can help.

 LIFESAVERS

- DVT (See DVT, page 100) is potentially life threatening. To decrease
your risk: drink lots of water and minimize coffee and alcohol to
prevent dehydration; request an aisle or bulkhead seat; walk the
aisles or stretch; and wear loose-fitting clothing and elastic compression stockings. If you are at high risk, take an aspirin (with food)
four hours before flying.

 TRIPSAVERS

- No Jet Lag is a combination homeopathic medicine that works
wonders for some travelers. Use at take-off, every two hours during
flight, and then each time you land. www.nojetlag.com

- JetZone is another combination homeopathic formula, more

similar to what we might put together, if you don't want single medicines. www.antijetlag.com

- An herbal option is Flight Spray. www.flightspray.com

- Although reviews are mixed, consider a jet-lag diet. Day one: "Feast" on high-protein breakfast and lunch and high carb dinner. Day two: "Fast": smaller, low-calorie, low carb meals, such as fruits, veggies, and salads. Day three: Feast. Day of departure: Fast. When you arrive: Break your fast with a high protein meal.

LEG CRAMPS

Also known as charley horses. Painful muscle spasms of the calf or thigh.

 HOMEOPATHY

- *Calcarea carbonica* (Calcium carbonate): Calf, foot, and thigh cramps, worse in bed, after exertion or going uphill. Bone and joint pain worse cold weather.

- **Calcarea phosphorica** (Calcium phosphate): Leg cramps better rubbing, worse skiing or in the snow. Growing pains. Bone, teeth problems.

- *Cuprum* (Copper): Cramps in palms, calves, soles. Spasms and cramping anywhere in the body. Muscle twitching legs. Jerking hands and feet.

 PREVENTION

- Stretch your leg muscles before and after physical activities.

- Drink plenty of fluids, especially in hot weather.

 MORE NATURAL TIPS

- Massage the affected limb towards the heart.

- Apply firm rotary pressure with thumb or forefinger to any tender points in the area until the tenderness decreases by half.

- Apply a hot pack or heating pad to the area to help relax the muscles.

- Take a hot bath with one cup of Epsom salt dissolved in the tub.

- Calcium 1500mg/day and Magnesium 500mg/day.

- For severe cramps after working or exercising in the heat, drink lightly salted water or take two salt tablets while drinking fluids to restore sodium and fluid lost through excessive sweating. Or drink electrolyte replacement liquids or V-8 juice.

TRIPSAVERS

- You don't want leg cramps on a red eye! Take Calcium and Magnesium as recommended above, drink lots of water on the plane, avoid alcohol and caffeine, and walk up and down the aisles before sacking out.

MALARIA

We include only a handful of tropical diseases in our book because there are many, you can research them online, and we have little experience treating them. But, the NUMBER ONE to consider is malaria! Every year 300-500 million cases occur worldwide, about 90% in sub-Saharan Africa, resulting in about two million deaths, mostly children. Drug-resistant strains are spreading and global warming is making the problem worse. If you are traveling to sub-Saharan Africa or one of the other areas of the world prone to malaria, you need to think ahead about what you want to do for prevention (See INSECT BITES AND STINGS, page 161). Malaria has been targeted by organizations such as the Gates Foundation because it is responsible for more fatalities than AIDS and TB combined. If you are traveling to sub-Saharan Africa, parts of Asia, or other areas prone to malaria, prevention and a plan of action in case of infection are essential.

Malaria is a parasite transmitted by the *Anopheles* mosquito. The likelihood of your contracting the disease depends on where you are going, how

M

173

long you will be there, what time of year, and what preventive measures you take.

Symptoms: periodic high fevers, sweating, muscle and joint pain, chills, bloody stools, headache, anemia, jaundice, vomiting, seizures, and coma. Malaria often recurs.

HOMEOPATHY

- **Arsenicum album** (Arsenic): Intense fever with burning heat. Exhausted, pale. Unquenchable thirst for sips. Clean tongue. Anxious, restless. Cold.

- **China** (Peruvian bark, the source of quinine): Periodic fevers. Chill, sweating, headache, nausea, weakness. Little thirst. Anxiety.

- *China sulphuricum* (Sulfate of quinine): Malaria with diarrhea and dysentery. Soft, large stools with rumbling in abdomen. Weakness from fluid loss.

- *Eupatorium perfoliatum* (Boneset): Bone pain as if they will break. Muscle soreness, vomiting, chill. Thirst and bitter vomiting. Pressure forehead.

- **Natrum muriaticum** (Sodium chloride): Violent headache. Chill begins at 10AM. Weak, short of breath, bone pain. Fever blisters lips. Great thirst.

Thankfully, we have not had to deal with malaria personally, and have treated only one patient for chronic malaria. For more specific information on the prevention and natural treatment of malaria, we recommend the informative travel book by our colleague, Richard Pitt, *The Natural Medicine Guide for Travel and Home*. He has lived in Africa and has much more experience than we do in this area (See BIBLIOGRAPHY, page 221).

Didi Ananda Ruchira, a homeopath in Kenya, developed a homeopathic protocol, used over the past 15 years with over 1500 Kenyan families, which she has found to be effective and affordable. We have not yet tried it ourselves, nor with patients. We are aware that this may be controversial, but feel it is worth sharing, given the widespread epidemic of malaria and the limited natural alternatives.

Didi's foundation, Abha Light recommends a 3-part program: 1) Start *Neem* 2X once a day. Continue for three weeks. For the first five days, while taking the *Neem*, add *China sulphuricum* 30C. On day 6, start MalariX, which contains *Malaria nosode, China, Natrum muriaticum, Arsenicum album*, and *Eupatorium perfoliatum.* Take 1 dose a day for 3 days, then 1 dose every 2 weeks. Continue taking MalariX every two weeks as long as the possibility of acquiring malaria exists. Didi has also found this combination to help prevent malaria. www.abhalight.org/malar.html

 PREVENTION

- Despite dire need, no effective vaccine is available. Efforts are ongoing.

- Anti-malarial medication, usually quinine-based, can cause undesirable side effects, and is not necessarily the prophylaxis of choice for those who live, work, or spend a lot of time in high-risk areas. They would have to spend much of their lives taking them. (See INSECT BITES AND STINGS, page 161 for further tips on how to not attract mosquitoes.)

- Stay inside when it is dark outside, preferably in a screened room with a fan or, even better, AC.

- Wear long-sleeved shirts and long pants.

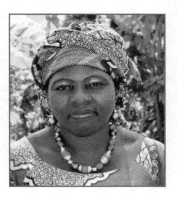

- Use mosquito repellants with DEET—use your judgment as to the strength. (See BUGS BE GONE, page 48). You can spray your outer clothing with permethrin before your arrival at the mosquito-prone destination, and use stronger repellants on your hands and other exposed areas.

M

- Use mosquito netting treated with permethrin.

- Avoid high-risk areas for mosquitoes and malaria if you are immune-compromised, pregnant, very young, or very old.

- If you are traveling to a high-risk malaria area, especially with your family, you may opt for conventional prophylaxis. But, if you will be exposed for six months or more, it is important to check out the side effects of the medications, along with longer-term effectiveness and cost. Two of the most common prophylactic medications are *Doxycycline* and *Mefloquine* (Larium). The longer you live in an area prone to malaria, the higher the risk of infection. You may be able to manage mosquito nets quite effectively for weeks, but the chances of a mishap increase after months or years. On the other hand, we just met an American public health doctor who travels to disaster spots worldwide on a moment's notice (she just returned from the brutal Philippines' typhoon). During her extended stays in Africa, she was meticulous about her mosquito net use, patching it whenever necessary, and never resorted to anti-malarial meds.

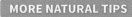

MORE NATURAL TIPS

- Artemisinin, made from the sweet wormwood plant, now rivals quinine drugs in terms of its rapid effectiveness with malaria. Wormwood has been used by Chinese herbalists for over 1500 years to treat malaria. Beware of the black-market version containing only chalk. Because of increasing Artemisinin resistance in the Mekong Delta countries of Thailand, Laos, Cambodia and Viet Nam, it is recommended to take Artemisinin in combination with another antimalarial (ACT therapy), selected to combat drug resistance in particular geographical areas to retain the effectiveness of Artemisinin therapy in malarial regions worldwide.

LIFESAVERS

- If you think you may have malaria, seek medical attention immediately.

TRIPSAVERS

- Before you plan your trip to Africa, Asia, or South/Central America, check out the malaria risk for your destination and plan accordingly, especially if traveling with small children, if you are elderly, or your immune system is compromised. There is great variability of risk from country to country, within countries, seasonally, and whether you are going to be urban or rural.

MEASLES

A viral illness affecting children and adults who do not have active immunity, it is highly contagious and spread by airborne droplets from an infected person *before* the rash appears and during the first few days of the illness. Symptoms include a fever up to 104F (40C), runny nose, sore throat, cough, light sensitivity, and an extensive, irregular, itchy rash. It starts around the ears, face, and neck, and lightens up as it spreads to the trunk and limbs as the fever decreases.

HOMEOPATHY

- **Aconite** (Monkshood): Take during first 24 hours of measles. First stage with sudden, high fever. Onset after exposure to cold dry air or wind. Bright, red, rough rash. Red eyes. Dry, barking, croupy cough. Itching, burning skin. Great restlessness.

- *Euphrasia* (Eyebright): Early stage. Eye symptoms are the chief complaint. Measles rash. Eyes light sensitive and water constantly.

- *Gelsemium* (Yellow jasmine): Beginning of measles with fever. Onset after fright or stage fright. Dizzy, drowsy, droopy, and dull. Muscle aches. Irritating watery nasal discharge. Hard, barky, croupy cough.

- *Pulsatilla* (Windflower): Later stage when fever is not high. Rash is dusky and beginning to fade. Runny nose and eyes with thick, yellow-green discharge. Earache or diarrhea as complication.

M

Not thirsty. Clingy.

- *Sulphur* (Sulfur): Measles rash late to appear. Lots of itching. Purplish, dusky skin. Itching worse from heat, in bed, and hot bath. Inflammation of eyelids with redness and burning.

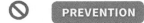

PREVENTION

- Some parents intentionally expose their children to measles when a neighbor or schoolmate becomes infected, so that it will not be a problem later in life. This is inconvenient just before leaving on a trip.

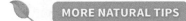

MORE NATURAL TIPS

- Bed rest in a darkened room.

- Drink lots of fluids and eat a light diet.

- Vitamin C 250mg twice a day for young children and 4 times if older. 1000mg 4 times a day for adults.

- Keep sores clean and avoid scratching.

- Oatmeal (1 cup finely ground to bath) or Aveeno baths for itching.

- To treat infected sores, apply a few drops of one part *Calendula* (marigold) tincture to 3 parts water. Cover with bandage or gauze.

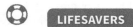

LIFESAVERS

- Do NOT give aspirin to a child with measles because they may develop Reye's syndrome, a brain and liver disease causing nausea, vomiting, mental dullness, memory loss, disorientation, and coma. Also, repeated exposure to Tylenol in childhood increases the risk of developing asthma.

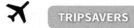

TRIPSAVERS

- Measles is highly contagious, so you will want to avoid exposure to an infected person prior to any planned travel.

MOTION SICKNESS (Travel Sickness)

You may be part of the third of the population prone to motion sickness. We speak from personal experience when we say that nothing can a ruin a trip faster than motion sickness, whether on the sea, in the air, or on land. We will never forget our infamous Molokini snorkeling trip, during a homeopathic conference on Maui, in Hawaii. A dozen seasoned homeopaths and not a single homeopathic medicine onboard as our boat heaved in the choppy water! The ginger ale recommended by the captain just didn't cut it. **Judyth:** I, along with a few other miserable homeopathic sailors, was heaving over the side of the boat. We mean it when we tell you not to leave home without your homeopathic kit. Although motion sickness will generally disappear after a few days, these recommendations can save you a lot of suffering in the meantime.

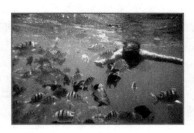

HOMEOPATHY

Homeopathy is great for motion sickness because, in addition to being highly effective, it does not cause the drowsiness and dryness of mouth of conventional medications, oral or patches, which may, in some cases, be vomited just when most needed.

- **Cocculus** (Indian cockle): Motion sickness with dizziness. Nausea from looking at moving objects out of the window of a moving vehicle. Must lie down. Worse from loss of sleep from caring for a sick loved one, and from the sight or smell of food.

- *Petroleum* (Coal oil): Motion sickness with a feeling of great emptiness in the stomach. Disorientation. Nausea from hunger. Heartburn. Dry, cracked skin. Relief from constant eating. Internal coldness. Better from warmth.

- **Tabacum** (Tobacco): Have you ever felt absolutely green, as if you had just smoked your very first cigarette? Think *Tabacum*. Deathly nausea. Worse from the least motion. Violent retching. Cold,

179

clammy, and pale. Spitting. Better from cold, fresh air and from opening the eyes.

PREVENTION

- Either drive or sit in the front seat of the car and look at distant objects or at scenery. Avoid reading. Distract yourself with music.

- On boats, trains, buses, cars, face forward and sit near a window.

- Keep your head as still as possible, by either bracing it, if seated, or lying semi-reclined.

- Go up on the deck of a boat, pick a point on the horizon, and hold a steady gaze. Choose a cabin in the middle of the ship, as close as possible to the waterline.

- In an airplane, choose a center or window seat over the wings where motion seem the least, and converse with your seatmate.

- In a car or boat, get plenty of fresh air.

- If sensitive, avoid strong smells such as tobacco smoke or gasoline.

- Eat lightly before traveling, and avoid alcohol, spicy, greasy, or heavy foods. Saltine crackers may alleviate nausea.

- Drink minimally unless you become dehydrated.

- Take your preferred medicine, herb, or medication BEFORE you travel.

MORE NATURAL TIPS

- Ginger, in the form of ale, capsules, candy, powder, or oil can relieve nausea. Use just before preventively as well as frequently during travel.

- Sip flat Coca cola (we include this in the natural category because the original *Coke* recipe, in 1885, did contain both coca leaves and kola nuts). Bob's mom used to give him Coke syrup, as a child, to settle his stomach. It is still sold by some pharmacies over the counter.

- Ski sickness is a form of motion sickness affecting skiers in heavy fog with poor visibility. (Nausea, dizziness, headache, fear of heights). Try homeopathic *Borax*, known for helping fear of downward motion.

- Wrist acupressure bands for motion sickness are widely available.

- If vomiting or loss of balance is severe, see a doctor immediately.

- Do NOT drive a vehicle if you are extremely dizzy, drowsy, disoriented, or ill.

LIFESAVERS

- Motion sickness could only be fatal if you were incapacitated by it while piloting a plane or steering a boat or other vehicle, which would be highly unlikely. The following precautions are to avoid serious health risk while flying.

- Travelers with severe heart conditions, such as unstable angina, congestive heart failure, or a recent heart attack or stroke, are best to postpone air travel, if possible. Those with serious lung conditions including acute asthma and emphysema should also think twice before flying. Supplemental oxygen, if needed, must be arranged ahead of time and provided by the airline.

- Pregnant women may not be allowed on some international flights after 36 weeks of gestation. You may need a medical letter documenting your due date. An uncomplicated delivery could be handled on board, but best not to take the chance, even if permitted. A challenging dilemma: Is the place of birth the registered country of the airline? Point of desembarkation? International airspace?

- Anemia: Anyone whose hemoglobin is less than 8.5 is safest not to fly.

- Scuba divers who fly in a low-pressure environment too soon after diving risk decompression illness.

TRIPSAVERS

- **Judyth:** I love to be on the water, but I am prone to seasickness. I have been saved, more times than I could count, by the Paihia

M

Bomb, which we discovered a decade ago in the Bay of Islands, New Zealand. It consists of two capsules, an antihistamine taken an hour before travel, followed by a caffeine pill taken an hour later. Savvy sailors worldwide order it by phone, without a prescription, from the Paihia Pharmacy (64 09-402 7034). Thanks to the bomb, I was able to enjoy a dolphin-watch cruise on the north coast of New Zealand, and a cruise on the *Navimag* ferry in southern Patagonia, while many around me were retching miserably.

MUMPS

This contagious viral infection of the parotid gland in the upper jaw, just below and in front of the ears and salivary glands, usually occurs in children but can be more serious in adults. It presents with high fever, chills, painful swelling of the parotid glands and other salivary glands, fatigue, and loss of appetite.

HOMEOPATHY

- *Abrotanum* (Lady's love): Inflammation of the testes after mumps. The parotid gland swelling goes down and the testes begin to swell.

- *Carbo vegetabilis* (Charcoal): Swollen, inflamed parotid glands. After becoming chilled, mumps go to the testes or breasts, which become swollen and inflamed. Bloating, gas, belching, exhaustion. Chilly but wants to be fanned.

- *Jaborandi* (Pilocarpus jaborandi): Mumps with increased sweating and salivation. Parotid glands double their usual size. Flushed face. Throat dry and inflamed. Inflammation of the testes after mumps.

- *Mercurius* (Mercury): Swollen, painful parotid gland. Increased salivation with bad breath, bad or metallic taste in mouth, and heavily coated tongue. Chilly, sweaty. Aggravated by both heat and cold. Worse night.

- **Phytolacca** (Pokeroot): Parotid gland swollen, tender, and stony

M

hard. Pain extends to the ear on swallowing. Swollen lymph nodes neck and behind ear.

- *Pulsatilla* (Windflower): Swollen, inflamed, painful parotid glands. Enormously swollen testes in boys and swelling of breasts in girls after mumps. Dry mouth without thirst. Worse hot, stuffy room. Wants air.

PREVENTION

- Isolate the person with mumps to avoid contagion.

- A very small percentage of those receiving a second dose of the MMR vaccine still contract mumps.

MORE NATURAL TIPS

- Rest.

- Eat soft foods to reduce the need for chewing.

- Avoid spicy, sour foods and drinks, which may stimulate salivary glands.

- Vitamin C 500mg two times a day for children four years or older and 1000mg 4 times a day for adults.

- Warm or cold packs to the swollen, inflamed salivary glands may help.

- Carrot poultice: Grate 2-3 carrots. Place in a cloth or cheesecloth and apply under chin for 2-8 hours. Cover with plastic to avoid staining.

M

LIFESAVERS

- There are four serious complications of mumps: meningitis, encephalitis, deafness, and orchitis (infection of the testicles). All may occur without the classic parotid swelling. Most children/adults recover fully.

- Do NOT give aspirin to a child with mumps because they may develop Reye's syndrome, a potentially life-threatening brain and liver disease causing nausea, vomiting, mental dullness, memory loss, disorientation, and coma.

- Those infected are considered contagious for five days after the glands begin to swell. The chance of catching mumps on a plane is small.

NAUSEA AND VOMITING (See Food Poisoning, Motion Sickness)

These symptoms can be triggered by many factors, including strong odors, morning sickness, motion sickness, food poisoning, indigestion, intestinal obstruction, alcohol intoxication and drug use, anxiety, and fright.

HOMEOPATHY

- *Bismuth* (Bismuth): Desire for cold water, which is vomited as soon as it reaches the stomach. Vomits more liquids than solid foods. Stomach pain, burning, and cramping. Pain feels like a heavy load in one spot. Clingy.

- ***Ipecac.*** (Ipecac root): Terrible, constant nausea not better from vomiting. First remedy for vomiting. Hates eating or smelling food. Tongue is clean. Bleeding along with nausea. Not thirsty.

- *Nux vomica* (Quaker buttons): Nausea and vomiting from anger and frustration. Straining to vomit, but can't. Violent vomiting. Wakes 3AM.

- *Phosphorus*: Vomits blood like coffee grounds. Stomach pain relieved by cold drinks. Great thirst for cold drinks, which help, but are vomited after becoming warm in the stomach. Wants fizzy drinks and company.

- ***Tabacum*** (Tobacco): Deathly nausea. Feels wretched. Violent vomiting from the least motion. Spitting with nausea. Cold, clammy, pale. Better fresh air.

- ***Veratrum album*** (White hellebore): Violent vomiting and diarrhea. Projectile vomiting. Icy cold with cold sweat on forehead while vomiting. Desires ice, cold drinks, sour, juicy fruit, and salt.

PREVENTION

- Avoid foods that are hard to digest.
- If the smell of hot food makes you sick, eat cool or cold meals.
- Eat smaller meals with less rich food.
- Rest after eating, with your head higher than your feet.
- If you wake up nauseated, keep crackers by the bed and eat on waking.
- You may want to avoid drinking during meals.
- Drink at least six glasses of water a day.
- Avoid acidic drinks like orange or grapefruit juice.
- Popsicles or iced drinks may prevent vomiting.

MORE NATURAL TIPS

- Get fresh air.
- Eat small amounts of food frequently.
- Crackers, tea, and toast may help.
- Eat bland foods.
- Drink clear fluids if you can keep them down.
- Sip ginger root tea, eat dried ginger, or drink ginger ale.
- Stimulate Stomach 36, an acupressure point in the soft place below the knee, to the outside of the leg where the tibia and fibula bones meet.

LIFESAVERS

- Push fluids!! If you are out in the middle of nowhere and have persistent vomiting, avoid dehydration, or you may end up in the hospital. Babies can die quickly from vomiting- or diarrhea-induced dehydration.

TRIPSAVERS

- If cigarette smoke makes you sick, eat outdoors, choose tables in non-smoking sections, if available, sit by opening windows wherever possible. Fortunately, smoking in restaurants, and other public buildings, is now prohibited in many countries of the world. We remember clearly when the inside of planes reeked of cigarettes. In those days, we always requested "no smoking seats," which sometimes meant smokers in the row directly behind us! If really ill, summon your courage to ask the smokers to please refrain. The worst they can do is to look at you like you are crazy and to refuse. Try homeopathic *Tabacum* for nausea after exposure to tobacco smoke.

NOSEBLEEDS

They may be caused by nasal infection, dry or cracked nasal mucous membranes, ruptured blood vessels and trauma, and vigorous nose-picking.

HOMEOPATHY

- *Arnica* (Leopard's bane): Nosebleed after an accident, traumatic injury, washing the face, or a fit of coughing.

- **Belladonna** (Deadly nightshade): Sudden nosebleed. Nosebleed with a red, dry, flushed face and glassy eyes. Very sensitive to light, noise, jar.

- **Ferrum phosphoricum** (Iron phosphate): Nosebleeds in children. Flushed face, red cheeks or pale face. Profuse bright red blood that clots easily.

- *Hamamelis* (Witch hazel): Profuse, slow nosebleed without clots. Dark red blood. Weak veins in nose. Hemorrhoids with nosebleeds.

- *Lachesis* (Bushmaster snake): Nosebleeds on left side with dark blood. Decrease when menstrual flow begins. Feels pressure inside the nose.

- **Phosphorus**: Profuse bright red blood. Doesn't clot. Bleeds easily. Better lying on the right side. Very thirsty for cold, fizzy drinks.

PREVENTION

- Use saline nose drops or spray.

- Avoid blowing your nose forcefully.

- Don't pick your nose or remove crusts.

- Avoid lifting or straining after a nosebleed.

- Elevate your head while sleeping.

- Apply a moisturizing salve or ointment to the inside of your nostrils.

- Avoid antihistamines or decongestants, which dry mucous membranes.

- Do not smoke.

- Do not use cocaine or amphetamines.

- Maintain normal blood pressure.

MORE NATURAL TIPS

- Apply direct pressure by squeezing sides of nose shut with thumb and forefinger for 5-10 minutes while breathing through mouth.

- Put a small piece of ice under upper lip beneath nose.

- Apply pressure to the point just under nose on upper lip.

- Apply a cold compress to the nose.

P

PINWORMS

These are tiny, white worms that come out of the anus of young children, most frequently from 5 to 10 years of age. The main symptom is itching, but the condition has been associated with appendicitis, convulsions, abdominal pain, and insomnia.

HOMEOPATHY

- **Cina** (Wormseed): Intense itching around anus with scratching. Also in nose—bores finger into nose to scratch. Grinds teeth. Irritable, defiant.

- *Ratanhia* (Krameria): Pinworms and anal fissures. Anus dry, itchy, burning, like splinters of glass. Intense rectal itching.

- *Sabadilla* (Mexican grass): Pinworms and hay fever with violent, fitful sneezing and runny nose. Sensation of crawling and itching in rectum.

- *Silica* (Flint): Pinworms. Constipation with rabbit-pellet stools.

- **Spigelia** (Pinkroot): Pinworms. Crawling and itching in anus. Twitching.

- *Teucrium* (Cat thyme): Pinworms. Itchy anus prevents sleep.

- *Urtica urens* (Stinging nettle): Intense burning, stinging, and itching around anus. Pinworms and hives.

PREVENTION

- Wash hands with soap and warm water after going to the bathroom and before eating.

- Avoid scratching the anus.

- Keep fingernails short and clean.

- Washing bedding and pajamas regularly, using a hot clothes dryer. Do NOT shake out before placing in the wash machine.

- Make sure your child puts on clean underwear every morning.

- Vacuum your child's play area frequently.

P

MORE NATURAL TIPS

- The Scotch Tape test is the quick and dirty way to diagnose. Place a piece of Scotch Tape over the anus at night, and look for worms or eggs on the tape in the morning. The definitive diagnosis is to have the tape examined under a microscope.

- If infected, bathe every morning to remove as many eggs as possible. Showering is best so as not to contaminate the bath water.

- We recommend using homeopathy first, before resorting to a pharmaceutical anti-parasitic drug. We have found it to be very effective, and much safer than conventional medication, which may have to be used repeatedly for re-infections. Be especially cautious in children under the age of two. If you do go the pharmaceutical route and expense is a concern, get Reese's Pinworm Medicine over the counter, which is apparently as effective.

- Garlic—eat raw, add to food, or make a salve and apply to rectum. Can kill eggs and relieve itching. http://www.thesnapmom.com/goot-natural-salve-treatment/

- In India locals use 1 T. fresh grated coconut followed by 1 t. castor oil three days later. Repeat once a day until pinworms are gone.

- We do not recommend worm-killing herbs like wormwood, even though they are effective, because they are so strong. We know because we used to put wormwood powder around the veggie garden to kill slugs.

POISON IVY, OAK, AND SUMAC (Contact Dermatitis)

P

Poison ivy is the world's most common allergy, affecting nearly half of the U.S. population. Each year about 50 million people suffer from reactions to poison ivy, oak, and sumac—including many who do not have other allergies. The eruptions are itchy, red, blistering, and quite annoying.

HOMEOPATHY

- *Anacardium* (Marking nut): Blistering eruption, especially face, hands, fingers. Yellow discharge oozes from blisters and crusts over. Scratches to the point of bleeding, but scratching makes the itching much worse.

- *Croton tiglium* (Croton oil): Incredible itching. Skin is dry and hard. Rash worst on face and genitals. Skin feels very tight. Scratching is painful. May have gushing diarrhea along with skin rash.

- *Rhus tox.* (Poison ivy): First remedy for poison ivy or similar rashes. Water-filled blisters. Intense itching. Restlessness. Stiff joints.

PREVENTION

- Learn what poison ivy, oak and sumac plants look like and AVOID them!

- Do not touch your pet's fur if the animal has contacted these plants.

- Do NOT burn poison ivy—it can go to your lungs and be very uncomfortable.

MORE NATURAL TIPS

- To remove the plant oil (urushiol), first use a solvent that can separate the oil from your skin surface, such as rubbing alcohol. Then rinse well with water. If you have no solvent, rinse well in water right after exposure.

- A poison ivy rash develops 1-2 days after exposure. At that point, soothe the skin, protect it from infection and spreading, and help blisters heal.

- Be careful NOT to scratch because it can make the rash spread.

- Wash the area with mild soap and water. Cover with sterile gauze. Keep clean.

- *Calendula* (marigold) lotion can soothe the rash and irritated skin.

- Calamine lotion can reduce itching. Dilute with water if it burns.

- For children, avoid combination topical products used along with antihistamines because, in excess, they can be absorbed through the skin.

- A compress with full-fat, ice-cold milk can help dry the rash and soothe the itch.

- Try cold, wet applications of water or comfrey root tea.

- Milk of magnesia may help topically due to its alkalinity.

- Take an oatmeal bath with 1 c. finely ground, dry oatmeal in the tub, or Aveeno.

- For secondary infections from scratching, use *Calendula* lotion, diluted tincture, or gel or topical colloidal silver.

- If you run into poison oak and mugwort (*Artemesia vulgaris*) is growing next to it, rub over the area of contact. It is reputed to neutralize the effect.

 TRIPSAVERS

- If you are going to an area known for poison ivy and its relatives, in a pinch, follow the recommendation of the U.S. Forestry Service: Use a spray deodorant on your arms and legs. Ironically, it is the aluminum chlorohydrate that prevents urushiol from getting into your skin (we normally avoid aluminum-containing products). Don't use on your face.

- The fastest, cheapest treatment to temporarily soothe itching and discomfort is plain ice for one minute. Do not use with blisters or weeping. Then use homeopathy for deeper healing.

POLIO

Polio is a highly contagious, historically devastating disease that has been basically eliminated in the Western hemisphere in the second half of the 20th century by immunization campaigns. Harrowing films of victims in iron lung machines are more than enough to strike fear in those resistant to immunization for this disease. Polio, still endemic in Pakistan, Afghanistan, and Nigeria, mainly affects children under the age of 5. Irreversible paralysis of the legs or lungs occurs in only 1 case in 200. It begins with flu-like symptoms (cold, fever, sore throat, cough).

P

 HOMEOPATHY

- **Lathyrus** (Chickpea): The #1 medicine. Spasticity and rigidity of legs. Knee jerks. Stiffness of ankles and knees with limping. Lower

191

limbs emaciated. Dragging gait. Infantile paralysis.

- *Cuprum* (Copper), *Silica* (Flint), and *Plumbum* (Lead) have been mentioned in the homeopathic literature, but *Lathyrus* is best known.

 PREVENTION

- Polio occurs in areas of inadequate sanitation and hygiene.

- The CDC (Center for Disease Control and Prevention) recommends a series of vaccines, from the age of two months. www.cdc.gov/vaccines/vpd-vac/polio/in-short-both.htm The dead form of the polio vaccine has eliminated the problem of viral shedding, which was a problem with the previously prevalent live polio vaccines. We advise parents to investigate for themselves the pros and cons of each vaccine, including polio. Administering a number of vaccines at the same time, or to children who are at all immune compromised, is not recommended.

- Dr. John Bastyr, the namesake of Judyth's naturopathic college, and an icon in naturopathic medicine, administered *Lathyrus* prophylactically in the 1950s, in Seattle, to over 5,000 patients, none of which contracted the disease. Some homeopaths recommend one dose of *Lathyrus* 200C before visiting an endemic area, then once a week if there is continued threat or exposure. Others suggest *Lathyrus* 30C once a month for prevention. It is a hot topic of debate among homeopathic skeptics, and we have no personal or clinical experience on which to comment. To decide for yourself, read *The Weight of Evidence: Homeopathy in Times of Epidemic and Related Statistics* by Andre Saine, N.D.

 LIFESAVERS

- Though rare, heads up if traveling in polio-endemic areas. The virus can cause total paralysis within hours. Among those paralyzed, 5%-10% die when their respiratory muscles become immobilized. If you have any suspicion of having contracted polio, seek immediate emergency care.

SCIATICA

This pain, along the distribution of the sciatic nerve in the back of the leg, results from inflammation and compression of the nerve root near the spine, or in the buttocks or pelvis. It may result from a herniated disk. The pain starts in the back and radiates down as far as the foot. There can also be numbness and tingling. Pain can be worse from sneezing, coughing, or straining.

HOMEOPATHY

- *Agaricus* (Fly agaric): Severe sciatica and low back pain. Muscle spasms, twitching, tension, tremor. Shooting and burning pain along the spine.

- *Colocynthis* (Bitter cucumber): Sciatica after anger, insult, or offense. Cramps in hips and thighs. Worse motion and right side. Better lying on the painful side or bending double.

- **Hypericum** (St. John's wort): Sciatic injury causing sharp, cutting pains along nerve. Shooting sciatic pain after injury to the spine or tailbone.

- *Lachesis* (Bushmaster snake): Right-sided (unlike other *Lachesis* symptoms, which are worse on the left side). Skin very sensitive. Feeling of pressure inside leg.

- **Rhus tox.** (Poison ivy): Sciatica from overexertion or sitting too long. Stiffness is the main symptom. Wants to stretch, move, or change position. Extreme pain on rising from sitting. Better hot bath, worse cold, damp.

PREVENTION

- Lift heavy loads carefully, keeping back straight and using leg muscles.

- Yoga exercises, with an experienced instructor, can stretch your back muscles and make injury less likely. Use along with back and abdominal strengthening exercises.

S

- Lose weight if you are carrying around more pounds than you need.
- Weak abdominal muscles may predispose to an increased risk of sciatica. Pilates will work wonders to strengthen your core and powerhouse!

MORE NATURAL TIPS

- Resume normal activity as soon as possible, rather than bed rest.
- Sleep well in a comfortable bed.
- Avoid strain or excessive stretching.
- Avoid intense exercise and physical activity, especially heavy lifting and trunk twisting, if you have acute back pain.
- Apply heat locally. A heat wrap worn 8 hours a day may allow you to keep up with your normal travel pace, but don't overdo it.
- Alternating hot and cold packs, first hot for 3 minutes, then cold for one minute, repeat three times. Do 2-3 times a day.
- Take a hot bath with one cup of Epsom salt added.
- Eat a fresh, healthy, natural diet high in fruits and veggies and low in caffeine and alcohol.
- Take Calcium 1200mg and Magnesium 600mg a day for muscle spasms.
- Traumeel homeopathic ointment can be quite helpful.
- We use a natural anti-inflammatory that contains bromelain, turmeric, and quercetin (a bioflavonoid).

TRIPSAVERS

- If prone to lower back problems, do NOT lift heavy luggage. Pack light. Use lightweight, wheeling bags. Avoid heavy backpacks. Get help lifting.
- Choose your seat wisely on long plane flights. Try for aisle and bulkhead seats. Get help placing your carry on in the overhead compartment. Get up, when possible, and walk up and down the aisle. Do airplane yoga.

SHOCK (See Also Allergic Reactions for Anaphylactic Shock)

Shock results from inadequate blood and oxygen flow to organs and tissues due to trauma, blood loss, dehydration, or other causes. Shock is a MEDICAL EMERGENCY and can lead rapidly to death. Apply first aid measures (see LifeSavers below) and call 911 or the equivalent. Symptoms include dizziness, fainting, moist and clammy skin, irregular breathing, fast pulse, weakness, vomiting, and thirst. These can progress to unresponsiveness, in which case the eyes appear shrunken, skin blotchy, and body temperature plummets.

HOMEOPATHY

- **Aconite** (Monkshood): Shock where terror is prominent. Sudden symptoms. Violent heart palpitations, profuse sweating, rapid pulse. Extreme anxiety, restlessness, fear of impending death.

- **Arnica** (Leopard's bane): Shock after an accident or traumatic injury. Any kind of shock. Shock from blood loss of any kind. Fainting. Any trauma with bruising. Victim refuses help.

- *Camphora* (Camphor): Shock with collapse. Sudden loss of strength with barely perceptible pulse. Icy cold, but wants to be uncovered.

- **Carbo vegetabilis** (Charcoal): Shock with collapse, weakness, exhaustion, hard to breathe. Bluish lips, pale skin. Wants to be fanned.

- *China* (Peruvian bark): Shock from blood loss. Chills, weakness, sweat.

- *Veratrum album* (White hellebore): Collapse with bluish color, cold sweat, vomiting, diarrhea. Feels icy cold. Wants ice, cold drinks, sour.

PREVENTION

- To prevent electric shock: Always use three-prong plugs. Use Ground Fault Circuit Interruptors (GFCIs) whenever possible. Outdoor outlets need weatherproof covers. Never use an appliance with a frayed cord. Be aware of power line locations. Never touch or try to move a downed power line. Do not touch an electrocuted person directly—use a piece of wood, not your hand.

MORE NATURAL TIPS

- Use homeopathy only, in addition to the emergency measures, rather that administering any herbs or other natural treatments.

LIFESAVERS

- Keep the person warm. Cover with a blanket.

- If serious, put victim flat on back and elevate feet above heart.

- For minor shock, get victim into a seated position with head between knees.

- Loosen clothing at neck, waist, and wherever else it is binding.

- Stop blood loss with direct pressure.

- Check airway and breathing and give CPR if necessary.

- Do not give anything by mouth that must be swallowed (2-3 tiny homeopathic pellets can be put on the tongue or mixed with a few drops of water).

- Turn head to allow the person to vomit if needed.

- Move to shade if the victim is out in the direct sun.

- Mix 1 t. salt and 2 t. baking soda into a quart of room temperature water. Give ½ c. over 15 minutes unless vomiting.

- Immediate hospitalization with IV fluids, drugs, or surgery as needed.

SKIN INFECTIONS (Abscesses, Boils)

Symptoms include redness, heat, pain, swelling, tenderness, and fever. We were off on a Brazilian Amazonian adventure in the Mamirau Reserve, a boat trip away from Tefe, which is a plane trip from Manaus. The Reserve is situated in the middle of the jungle, surrounded by countless caimans (crocodiles), botos (pink river dolphins), and ua-karis (rare, red-faced, white haired monkeys). **Judyth:** Mosquitoes find me delectable, and the dusk canoe trips in search of the unusual creatures made me easy bait. In order to soothe the incessant itching, I bought a rough-hewn fish bone from a local artisan with the intention of turning it into a primitive skin scratcher. There was no source of reliable fresh water for bathing, the bites became infected, and I went home with the dreaded MRSA (antibiotic-resistant *Staph aureus*). No picnic! I did find a wonderful garlic product (see Allimed below) that cured the MRSA.

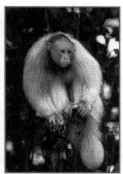
Uakari monkey

HOMEOPATHY

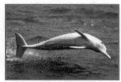
Boto pink river dolphin

- *Arsenicum album* (Arsenic): Pustules that are black or filled with blood. Small, red, ulcerated pimples with bad-smelling discharge. Burning pain.

- **Hepar sulphuris** (Calcium sulfide): Boils or abscesses that are exquisitely sensitive to pain, cold, touch. Splinter-like pains. Thick pus smells bad, rotten, or sour. Helps to expel foreign bodies from boils. Irritable.

- *Lachesis* (Bushmaster snake): Bluish purple or black abscess. Abscess feels better as soon as it drains. Worse left side.

- *Mercurius* (Mercury): Abscesses or ulcers. Bad-smelling pus. Boils are inflamed with burning, stinging pain and rapid formation of pus. Bad breath, increased saliva, offensive body odor. Worse from heat and cold.

- **Silica** (Flint): Infections from a foreign body or splinter. Has not yet drained. Boil is filled with bad-smelling pus. Lymph nodes hard and swollen. Abscess with bad-smelling pus. Infections slow to heal.

⊘ PREVENTION

- Wash hands often with clean, warm water and soap. Use an

alcohol-based sanitizer if there is no clean water available in order to prevent spread of infections.

- Clean and treat any skin lesions immediately. If hiking or in dirty environments, keep lesion covered.

- Avoid contact with others' infected lesions or towels.

- Avoid touching your eyes, nose, and mouth with your hands.

- Avoid using hot tubs and sharing baths if you have infected lesions.

MORE NATURAL TIPS

- If the abscess is draining, cover with gauze dressing and keep clean.

- Alternating hot (5 minutes) and cold (1 minute) compresses.

- Use massage techniques to promote lymphatic drainage.

- Hot, moist packs can be helpful for boils, to bring the infection to a head.

- Immune support: echinacea and goldenseal, elderberry, Reishi or other mushrooms.

- Colloidal silver or *Calendula* (marigold) tincture topically.

- Vitamin A 25,000 IU, Vitamin C 1000mg 3 times/ day, zinc 30-50mg/ day.

TRIPSAVERS

- If you are prone to skin infections, we highly recommend taking along one of the Allimed products (strong, highly-effective, garlic products). www.allimed.us

- If you are in a tropical area or away from civilization and you get a scratch, keep it clean, disinfect, and cover promptly. You don't want to end up in a foreign hospital with a *Staph* infection!

SNAKEBITES

Take heart: The risk of snakebite to travelers is very low. Snakes are generally not aggressive and will bite only when provoked. Only a small minority of snakes have venom that is dangerous to humans. Not all bites from poisonous snakes contain sufficient venom to cause a serious problem. If you are in a place near an urban hospital, it is very likely they will have anti-venom for the particular snake.

HOMEOPATHY

The very best homeopathic medicine to take is the one from the snake that bit you, but those below are the most common available. You can purchase other more unusual snake medicines from a homeopathic pharmacy.

- *Crotalus cascavella* (Brazilian rattlesnake): Bluish or reddish discoloration or spots. Bleeding from all orifices. Can only swallow liquids. Stringy, clotted bleeding. Feels as if someone is standing behind.

- *Crotalus horridus* (American rattlesnake): Swelling of body parts. Intolerance of clothing. Burning thirst for great quantities of cold water. Faintness during palpitations. Irritable.

- *Elaps* (Coral snake): Black discharges and hemorrhages. Right-sided paralysis. Cold drinks feel like ice in stomach. Crave salad, oranges, and ice. Dread of being alone or in the rain.

- *Lachesis* (Bushmaster snake): Bluish, purplish, or mottled discoloration of skin. Throbbing pain in veins. Intense pressure. Worse left side. All symptoms feel better after discharge. Lump in throat. Throat feels constricted. Even the slightest touch aggravates.

- *Naja* (Cobra): Less prone to hemorrhage. Constriction of body parts. Worse left side to right. Puffy hands, feet. Can't lie on left side. Cold.

- *Vipera* (Pit viper): Swollen blood vessels, especially veins. Heel pain better lifting foot. Bruised, blackish, mottled skin. Intolerance of clothing.

S

PREVENTION

- Do not walk in unknown areas without footwear and protective clothing. Walk on the paths, and use a flashlight at night. Outhouses are popular resting places for snakes.

- Snake-bite kits are controversial.

- If you meet a snake, remain still and it will likely retreat.

- Don't put your hands in holes in the ground, woodpiles, or under rocks.

- Don't swim in swamps or rivers with heavily matted vegetation.

- If in snake country, check your footwear, clothing, and corners of the room when you wake up in the morning.

MORE NATURAL TIPS

- Take along activated charcoal powder in capsule form or ground finely. Dampen powder and apply to the fang wounds as soon as possible. Keep firmly in place with a band-aid or tape. Then take 2 t. of wet charcoal internally. After the first 24 hours, activated charcoal won't work.

- Other options are Bentonite Clay powder, also made into a paste, or echinacea capsules. Apparently the derogatory term "snake oil" originated with echinacea because it was known to help snakebites. Take 4 capsules of Echinacea per hour for 4 hours, then 2 capsules every two hours, until the crisis is over.

LIFESAVERS

If you are bitten:

- Stay calm. Move the person away from the snake to avoid another bite.

- Immobilize the limb with a splint. Keep at or below heart level.

- Call for transport immediately to the nearest hospital.

- Clean the wound gently, and carefully to remove any excess venom.

- Remove the victim's jewelry and loosen clothing.

- Use a pen to mark any reddened or swollen area to monitor changes.

- Apply an Ace-type elastic bandage to the entire limb to slow venous and lymphatic flow. Make sure you can still feel a pulse away from the bandage closer to the hand or foot. Keep in place until reaching the hospital.

- If the snake is dead, take it along with you. If not, try to identify it.

- DO NOT run after the snake, even if decapitated, in rattlesnakes and other venomous snakes, the head may still bite reflexively for up to an hour afterwards!

- DO NOT cut the wound or try to suck out the venom.

- DO NOT apply ice, heat, or a tourniquet.

- DO NOT give aspirin.

 TRIPSAVERS

- If you are hiking or camping, especially with children, ask ahead of time if there are poisonous snakes in the area and take precautions.

SORE THROAT

 HOMEOPATHY

- *Aconite* (Monkshood): Very sore, hot, dry, red throat after exposure to a cold, dry wind. Sudden onset of sore throat with a high fever. Restless.

- **Apis** (Honeybee): Swollen, fiery red sore throat that burns, stings. Better cold drinks and worse solid, sour, hot food. Right-sided. Swollen uvula.

S

- **Belladonna** (Deadly nightshade): Red, hot, burning sore throat, worse right side. Sudden onset. Bright red, hot, dry face. High fever (102-105F or 39-40.5C) with sore throat. Tonsillitis. Strep throat.

- *Hepar sulphuris* (Calcium sulfide): Exquisitely sensitive, painful sore throat with splinter-like pain or a feeling of a fish bone stuck in throat. Caused by cold draft. Pus-filled blisters, abscess smells like old cheese.

- **Lachesis** (Bushmaster snake): Left-sided throat pain or moves left to right. Worse swallowing or tight clothes around neck. Lump in throat.

- **Lycopodium** (Club moss): Right-sided or moves right to left. Better warm or room temperature drinks, worse cold drinks.

- *Mercurius* (Mercury): Sore, burning throat with salivation, bad breath, and bad taste in mouth. Bad-smelling sweat. Ulcerated tonsils and throat. Constant desire to swallow. Brings up large lumps of mucus.

- *Phytolacca* (Pokeroot): Dark red or bluish sore, puffy throat. Swollen neck glands. Throat pain goes to ear on swallowing. Lump in throat.

PREVENTION

- We recommend immune support with echinacea, goldenseal, olive leaf, elderberry, Reishi and other mushrooms, and vitamin C at the very first sign of a scratchy throat. Our patients swear by Immune-a-Day and Olive Leaf Relief. www.healthyhomeopathy.com/shop Take every two hours. If you hit it hard at the very beginning, it will often not even turn into a sore throat.

- Using a neti pot to irrigate the sinuses may also nip it in the bud.

MORE NATURAL TIPS

- Gargle with warm salt water three times a day or 1 t. *Calendula* tincture in one cup of warm water.

- Slippery elm tea or lozenges.

- Suck on zinc lozenges.

- Take vitamin C 1000mg 4 times a day and zinc 30-50mg.
- Avoid dairy products and sweets.
- Drink 1-2 glasses of fresh carrot juice.

SPRAINS AND STRAINS

Sprains are usually not severe, but will get your attention to slow down. They usually respond quickly to homeopathy. If pain is severe and persists, get an X-ray to rule out a fracture.

Judyth: While still in naturopathic college, just beginning to study home-opathy, I was hurrying down the stairs to a meeting, and my ankle twisted beneath me. Unable to put pressure on my foot due to the sharp pain, I literally crawled upstairs to my homeopathic kit, took *Arnica*, and applied ice. Fifteen minutes later I was able to walk down the stairs, gingerly, and made it to my meeting just in time. I explained the situation, and was able to elevate my leg during the meeting. When the pain returned to a much lesser degree a few hours later, I took one more dose of *Arnica*. The ankle was fine by the next day.

HOMEOPATHY

- ***Arnica*** (Leopard's bane): Give FIRST for sprain or strain. Muscles feel sore, painful, bruised. Injuries from overexertion. Shock after injury.

- ***Bryonia*** (Hops): Stiffness and shooting pain in the joints. Pain worse from ANY movement, better when immobile.

- *Ledum* (Marsh tea): Injured area is cold to the touch and better from ice or cold applications. Desire to soak feet in cold or icy water.

- ***Rhus tox.*** (Poison ivy): Sprains, strains with stiffness and pain bet-ter from moving, stretching, flexing. Injury to tendons and muscles after overexertion. Restless. Joint cracking. Better hot bath, worse cold.

S

- *Ruta* (Rue): Injury to flexor tendons, joints, cartilage, periosteum (outer layer of bone). Injury to ankle, wrist. Bruised, sore, aching. Stiff, restless.

PREVENTION

- Avoid exercising or playing sports when tired or in pain.

- Be careful to avoid falling (proper shoes, caution on ice, walking stick).

- Wear good shoes that fit well. Replace athletic shoes as soon as the tread wears out or the heel wears down on one side.

- Ease into any fitness routine.

- Warm up and stretch before exercising.

MORE NATURAL TIPS

- RICE Therapy: REST—preferably no weight on injured area for 48 hours, crutches or a cane if necessary. Apply an ICE pack for 20 minutes at a time, 4-8 times a day, no longer, or you will risk cold injury or frostbite.

- COMPRESSION, using an elastic wrap. ELEVATION to decrease swelling.

- Soak in Epsom salt tub to reduce swelling.

- Use a natural anti-inflammatory, like turmeric, bromelain, or quercetin.

TRIPSAVERS

- **Judyth:** We were running, with our luggage, to catch a bus in Quito, Ecuador on the way to Otavalo. I felt and heard a snap in my right knee. I hobbled up the steps of the bus in agony, knowing I had damaged the knee. Two hours later, when we arrived at our hotel, I could not take even a step. We had planned to go to the famous Saturday market the following day, then spend a week with the Huaorani Indians a few days later, which involved walking around in very primitive, isolated areas. The only crutches we found didn't really fit. The market visit did take place, with the help of a wheelchair, courtesy of the local *Cruz Roja* (Red Cross), and my helpful husband. It was too late to cancel our Amazon journey. That night we met with a three-generation Yachac shaman, whom we had met several years earlier on our island in the U.S. That night I woke at 1AM, shocked that I could walk. We met with Don Joaquin Pineda again the following morning, Christmas Day, and he explained that he had done a healing ceremony for me that night. We were duly impressed. We completed our Amazon trip successfully, though I remained cautious with the knee.

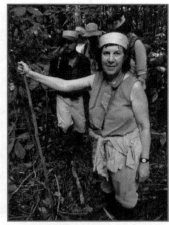

Hiking in the Ecuadorian Amazon with the Huaoranis

STOMACH ACHES AND ACUTE ABDOMINAL PAIN

GI pain can range from mild to incapacitating. Causes are highly variable, including indigestion, gas, appendicitis, gall bladder or liver problems, menstrual cramping, acute gastroenteritis, ectopic pregnancy, miscarriage, anxiety, and more serious diseases. Symptoms include localized or referred pain, cramping, nausea, vomiting, constipation, diarrhea, gas, bloating, abnormal stools, anxiety, rapid heartbeat and pulse, and sweating.

HOMEOPATHY

- **Bryonia** (Hops): Tenderness and throbbing just below stomach. Abdominal wall very tender. Stomach pains worse after eating or vomiting. Constipation with great dryness of rectum. Liver heavy, sore, and swollen. Severe abdominal pain. Appendicitis. WORSE MOTION.

S

205

- *Colocynthis* (Bitter cucumber): Violent, gripping, clutching pain in waves. Intestines feel squeezed between two stones. Drawing pains stomach. Pain better from hard pressure, doubling over, or bringing knees to chest. Colicky pain with gas. Symptoms after anger, indignation.

- *Cuprum* (Copper): Violent, cramping pains and spasms. Sudden stomach convulsions with vomiting. Abdominal cramping worse motion. Violent vomiting. Agonizing abdominal spasms and colic.

- *Dioscorea* (Wild yam): Unbearable, sharp, cutting, twisting, gripping pain that moves around suddenly. Worse doubling over; better standing erect. Gall bladder pain extending to the chest, back, arms.

- **Lycopodium** (Club moss): Sensation of a band around waist, worse from tight clothing and 4-8PM. Excessive, noisy gas. Bloating from least amount of food. Weak digestion. Right-sided. Better warm drinks.

- *Magnesia phosphorica* (Magnesium phosphate): Colicky pain with lots of gas. Abdominal pain radiating to both sides and back. Colicky pain radiating from navel. Must pass gas, loosen clothes, walk around. Better doubling over, rubbing, warmth, pressure, hot applications and drinks.

- **Nux vomica** (Quaker buttons): Stomach or abdominal pain after rich foods, alcohol. Violent vomiting. Sour burping. Constipation—no urge, Gallstone pain after anger. Worse eating. Better vomiting, hot drinks.

- **Pulsatilla** (Windflower): Heartburn or indigestion after fats, rich foods, pork, ice cream. Stomach feels heavy. Painful bloating with loud rumbling. Stools vary. Little thirst. Worse warm, stuffy room.

PREVENTION

- Eat lots of organic fresh fruits and vegetables, whole grains, nuts, seeds.

- Avoid fast food restaurants. Take your time and enjoy slow food instead.

- Do not overdo alcohol, caffeine, sweets, heavy, overly spicy, or rich foods.

- Do not eat or drink too quickly nor while doing something stressful.

- Drink only water with meals. Avoid pop, carbonated drinks with meals.

MORE NATURAL TIPS

- Charcoal absorbs gas. Take 2 caps every 2-4 hours as needed.

- Peppermint, fennel, or fenugreek tea can soothe stomach discomfort.

- Try castor oil packs applied for one hour with a heating pad. Lie on your back and bring knees to chest (wind-relieving pose).

LIFESAVERS

- If you develop severe pain in the middle of your abdomen that comes and goes, nausea and appetite loss, a mild fever, your right lower abdomen is tender to pressure, and you still have your appendix, see a doctor to rule out appendicitis. If not treated, it can turn into peritonitis, which can be fatal.

TRIPSAVERS

- Downing high calorie, non-nutritious food in a hurry is a recipe that will not make your digestive system feel content. Take delicious and nutritious snacks with you from home while traveling. Buy healthy meals or snacks in airports, train or bus stations, on airplanes or trains. Better to have bread/cheese or a wrap or salad, an apple or a banana, and bottled water rather than a greasy burger with French fries or a pizza.

STYES

Styes are an infection of a sweat or oil gland in the eyelid causing redness, swelling, tearing, and tenderness of the edge of the lid followed by a small, tender, hardened area. A chalazion is a scarring of the glands in the eyelids resulting from styes.

HOMEOPATHY

- *Hepar sulphuris* (Calcium sulfide): Eyelid is red, inflamed, pus-filled, and very sensitive. Inflammation and swelling of the eye with redness of sclera (white of eye). Little pimples around inflamed eye. Eyes tear and stick together at night due to secretion of hardened mucus. Eyes very painful in bright light. Chilly, irritable, hypersensitive to pain.

- *Lycopodium* (Club moss): Styes toward inner corner of eyelid, worse right eye. Redness of eyelid and sclera. Dryness and sticking pain. Eye goopy at night.

- **Pulsatilla** (Windflower): Lots of thick, yellow, bland discharge. Tearing, pain, and itching in eye better from cold applications. Feels something is covering the eyelid that needs rubbing away. Worse hot, stuffy room.

- **Staphysagria** (Stavesacre): Eyes dry or teary. Painfully inflamed sclera. Stinging pain inner corner of eyelid. Eyes dry on waking. Chronic styes.

- *Sulphur* (Sulfur): Eyes red during day and itch violently at night. Feeling of sand in the eye. Edge of eyelid red, irritated. Oily tears.

PREVENTION

- Keep eye cosmetic tools clean. Do not share cosmetics, other makeup tools, or face towels.

- Toss old or contaminated eye makeup.

- Do not touch the eyes. Wash your hands with warm water and soap before putting any drops or contacts in your eyes.

MORE NATURAL TIPS

- If you have conjunctivitis, keep the eyes clean, gently wipe off eyelids twice a day, and do not scratch itchy eyes or lids.

- Place compresses soaked in hot water on the eyelid 10 minutes several times a day to bring the stye to a head and allow it to drain.

- We use *Euphrasia* (Eyebright) herbal eye drops with our patients.

- Grated cucumber or potato poultices can reduce inflammation.

- Vitamin C 500mg 4 times a day.

- Add 1 cup of boiling water to a handful of fresh parsley. Steep 10 minutes. Soak a clean cloth and leave on eyes 15 minutes.

- Do NOT try to burst the stye. It could cause the infection to spread.

TRIPSAVERS

- We take along *Euphrasia* eye drops when we are in Chile, on the off chance of eye irritation or problems.

SUNSTROKE, HEATSTROKE, AND HEAT EXHAUSTION

Heatstroke, also called sunstroke, usually begins with a headache, dizziness, and fatigue leading to heat, flushing, and dryness of the skin, usually with scant perspiration. Breathing and pulse rates increase quickly, sometimes up to a pulse of 180 beats per minute; heat exhaustion, which is less severe, presents with gradual weakness, nausea, profuse perspiration, anxiety, and fainting. The skin is generally cold and clammy, the pulse weak, and blood pressure low.

HOMEOPATHY

- **Belladonna** (Deadly nightshade): Sudden, violent onset. Intense body heat. Throbbing or pounding headache, worse right side. Face bright red, hot, dry. Eyes glazed. Fullness and congestion of

S

blood to the head.

- ***Glonoine*** (Nitroglycerin): Quick onset of violent, throbbing headache. Blood rushes to the head. Bursting, expanding feeling in eyes, head, and organs. Worse from the sun, bright snow, the heat of a fire.

 PREVENTION

- Drink LOTS of cold water if working in the direct sunlight or humidity.

- Check to see how much water you need to pack if hiking or camping. Many visitors to the bottom of the Grand Canyon have died because they did not carry nearly enough water. If it seems like more than you can carry, hire a pack animal or skip the trip.

- Wear protective sun gear, dress cool in cool colors, wear sunglasses.

- If in very hot or humid climates, exercise before sunrise or after sunset.

- Older people, babies, young children, diabetics, and those who take antibiotics, are all particularly at high risk.

 MORE NATURAL TIPS

- If overheated, immediately take a cold shower or bath or wrap yourself in cold towels or ice.

- When hiking, take food not excessively salty (jerky, smoked fish, and salted nuts are all very high in sodium) to lessen the risk of dehydration.

- If extremely thirsty, don't drink water so quickly that you vomit.

- Coconut water is a great natural electrolyte solution. If in the tropics, this is easy to come by.

- Put 2 drops of peppermint oil on the back and sides of the neck, inside wrists, and on the soles of the feet to cool you down.

 LIFESAVERS

- Heatstroke (sunstroke) can progress to the point of disorientation, seizures, and unconsciousness. The body temperature can shoot up very quickly to 104F (40C), or even 106F (41C). In heatstroke, collapse of the heart can lead to permanent brain damage or death. This is a MEDICAL EMERGENCY. Before medical help arrives, try to cool down the person with an ice or cold pack on the top of the head and move out of the sun.

TRIPSAVERS

- Buy a set or two of long-sleeved, quick-wicking travel clothing and a hat that completely covers the back of your neck if going to areas of extreme sun.

- Carry a daypack with a hydration compartment plus any extra bottles of water needed. Carry a 5-gallon collapsible water container when hiking in areas without sources of fresh water, along with a filtration or purification device, or tablets.

TEETHING

Common symptoms are pain in the teeth and gums; drooling, redness, and swelling of the gums, fever, changes in BMs, restlessness, fussiness, difficulty sleeping.

HOMEOPATHY

- ***Calcarea carbonica*** (Calcium carbonate): Painful, delayed teething. Chubby babies with large heads who sweat on back of the head or neck during sleep. Tooth pain worse from cold air or hot food, drink.

- *Calcarea phosphorica* (Calcium phosphate): Teething and other problems with teeth and bones, such as fractures and growing pains. Teeth sensitive to chewing. Delayed, soft, easily-decayed. Fussy kids.

- ***Chamomilla*** (Chamomile): Fussy. Tantrums with kicking, hitting, and screaming during teething. Green diarrhea and ear infec-

T

tions during teething. Highly pain-sensitive. Inconsolable. Must be rocked or carried.

- *Silica* (Flint): Difficult, slow teething in delicate children who sweat. Gums painful, inflamed, swollen, worse from drinking cold water. Teeth break down quickly and decay or lose enamel. Dental abscesses.

MORE NATURAL TIPS

- Give the baby something cold to chew on: a pacifier or teething ring placed briefly in the freezer, ice, or cold, frozen washcloths.

- Mesh feeders with frozen bananas, mango, and other frozen fruit can soothe painful gums. Cut strings to 9" or less to prevent strangulation.

- Large, refrigerated or frozen pieces of carrot or celery that are cut too large to place entirely in the mouth.

- When cutting the first tooth, a finger can replace a plush chew toy.

- Old-fashioned, wooden teething toys/rings or wooden cooking spoon.

- Freeze as cubes: breast milk, diluted chamomile tea. Or ice slush.

TRIPSAVERS

- If you don't have *Chamomilla*, try Hyland's Teething Tablets, a low-potency combination homeopathic, or dilute chamomile tea. These may only work stopgap. A higher potency acts more deeply and lasts longer.

TOOTHACHE

Nerve pain can be very intense, even excruciating. So is the case with some dental pain. It may be worse chewing, eating or drinking hot and cold, and drafts. Common causes are tooth decay, dental abscess, nerve sensitivity, dental work, sinus infections, trauma, and damage to the facial nerve. If untreated, an infection of the teeth or gums can become systemic.

HOMEOPATHY

- **Chamomilla** (Chamomile): Violent toothache worse from coffee, warm food or drink, eating, entering a warm room. Hypersensitive to pain. Better cold drinks. Inconsolable with pain. Child screams with pain.

- **Coffea** (Unroasted coffee): Toothache relieved by holding cold water in mouth and worse as soon as it gets warm. Highly hypersensitive to pain, emotions.

- *Hepar sulphuri*s (Calcium sulfide): Toothache with abscess. Worse least draft. Hypersensitive to pain and drafts. Mouth smells like old cheese.

- **Mercurius** (Mercury): Tearing, shooting, or throbbing pains in decayed teeth or roots. Toothache extends to ears, cheek. Bad breath and bad or metallic taste in mouth. Drooling. Coated tongue.

- *Plantago* (Plantain): Unbearable, severe toothache worse from touch and extremes of hot or cold. Shoots up left side of face. Teeth sensitive and sore. Piercing, digging, violent tooth pain. Profuse salivation.

PREVENTION

- Don't allow babies to nurse continuously.

- Don't nurse the baby to sleep.

- Don't give a bottle with milk, formula, or juice before napping or sleep.

- Between feedings or at naptime, give a bottle of cold water to suck on.

- Keep the pacifier clean.

- Do NOT feed the baby sugar or pop, nor dip a pacifier in honey or sugar.

- Don't let your child continue thumb sucking past the age of four.

T

- Teach and reinforce good dental hygiene with your children.

- Teach family members and caregivers to give healthy snacks to your baby rather than decay-causing sweets.

- Practice good, regular dental hygiene, including brushing for at least two minutes, and flossing or irrigating, especially at night.

- Get regular dental cleanings and exams, have problems attended to promptly.

MORE NATURAL TIPS

- Ice may temporarily numb the pain.

- Clove oil applied to the gums is an effective pain reliever.

- Garlic decreases bacteria and pain. Apply a clove of crushed garlic directly on the affected tooth or take a garlic supplement high in allicin. www.allimed.us

TRIPSAVERS

- Keep up a healthy dental care routine even while traveling. We carry a small, battery operated irrigator with us.

- If dental pain arises during your travels, see a local dentist sooner rather than later. Dental treatment may not be your favorite pastime, but it is far better than ending up in the middle of nowhere in agony.

TYPHOID

Typhoid fever is caused by the *Salmonella typhi* bacteria and spread by contaminated food, drink, or water. They travel into your gut, through the bloodstream, then to your lymph nodes, gallbladder, liver, spleen, etc. It is common in developing countries. Symptoms begin with fever, malaise, and abdominal pain, and can progress (after 10-14 days) to bloody stools, chills, fatigue, weakness, confusion, and delirium. It can take 2-4 weeks to notice improvement.

A close friend contracted typhoid from drinking fruit juice from a street vendor in India. He became quite ill and the recovery was prolonged—a painful and uncomfortable cautionary tale.

HOMEOPATHY

- *Arnica* (Leopard's bane): Bruises, bedsores. Bruised feeling. Stupor. Is not aware of being sick. Involuntary stools and urine.

- *Arsenicum album* (Arsenic): Exhaustion with anxiety, restlessness. Dark, bad-smelling diarrhea, high fever. Thirst for sips of water. Worse after midnight.

- **Baptisia** (Indigo): Black or brownish coated tongue. Drowsy, dull. Blood poisoning. Feels bruised all over. Restless. Eyes heavy. High fever.

- *Bryonia* (Hops): Great soreness all over body. Fatigued. Does not want to move body. Is very thirsty for large quantities of water.

- *Gelsemium* (Yellow jasmine): Mild cases. Sore, bruised. Dull. Droopy eyelids. Little thirst. Lack of worry about the condition.

- *Manganum* (Manganese): Mild typhoid, after fever is gone, with sensitive, sore bones and slow recovery.

- *Rhus tox* (Poison ivy): Yellow-brown, bad-smelling diarrhea. Severe backache. Red-tipped tongue, very restless. Mutters, delirious.

PREVENTION

- Drink bottled or boiled water.

- If you are traveling to a high-risk area, consider the vaccine, at least one week before travel, though it's not always completely effective.

- Tuck electrolyte packets or Emergen-C in your luggage, just in case.

- Wash your hands well with warm water and soap before eating and after using the bathroom.

- If you are eating from a roadside stall, stick to foods that have been thoroughly cooked and are still hot and steaming.

- Ask for drinks without ice. Avoid popsicles and slushies.
- Avoid raw veggies and fruits that can't be peeled, especially salads.
- When peeling them, wash your hands well, peel them yourself, and toss the peels.

 MORE NATURAL TIPS

- Eat small meals often, especially high-protein and low-fiber.
- Drink lots of fluids and replace electrolytes.
- Avoid fried, fatty, spicy food. Eat bland and soft.

 LIFESAVERS

- Possible complications include severe GI bleeding, peritonitis, and kidney failure.

 TRIPSAVERS

- No matter how hot and parched you may be, do not even consider buying a refreshing, cold drink, other than out of a bottle, on the street.

VAGINAL INFECTION (Bacterial Vaginosis)

Common symptoms are redness of the vulva, itching, swelling, and pain of vulva, labia, and vagina.

 HOMEOPATHY

- *Caladium* (American arum): Terrible vaginal itching, worse during pregnancy. Dryness and burning of labia and vulva.
- *Kreosotum* (Creosote): Terribly itchy, burning, swelling. Acrid, yellow discharge. Extreme rawness. Worse scratches, before period.

- **Pulsatilla** (Windflower): Thick, bland, yellow-green discharge or milky, creamy and irritating. Weepy, moody. Not thirsty.
- **Sepia** (Cuttlefish ink): Discharge makes area feel raw, burning, itching. White or yellow, slimy, lumpy or bloody discharge. Worse during the day, before menses, during menopause. Aversion to sex. Irritable.

PREVENTION

- Avoid using harsh soaps, cleansers, body scrubs.
- Shower rather than taking a hot bath, which can cause vaginal irritation.
- If you do take a bath, rinse any soap away from the genital area.
- In general, avoid douches (except for the instructions below).
- Buy unscented menstrual pads or tampons.
- Wear cotton underwear rather than synthetic.
- Skip pants that are tight around the crotch.
- Avoid unprotected sex with new or multiple partners.

MORE NATURAL TIPS

- Insert one boric acid capsule vaginally in the morning and one acidophilus capsule at bedtime for 5 days (not during period).
- An alternative is a douche of 1 T. boric acid or half a cup of hydrogen peroxide to 2 quarts of warm water.
- For yeast vaginitis only on the labia and vulva, apply diluted vinegar mixed 1:1 with water topically or dilute grapefruit seed extract.
- *Calendula* (Marigold) cream can be very soothing topically to the vulva.
- We use, with patients, natural vaginal suppositories: vitamin E for vaginal dryness and *Calendula* herbal suppositories for vaginal infections.

TRIPSAVERS

- If you do develop a vaginal infection during your trip, deal with it then rather than waiting. Bacterial vaginosis may lead to a number of complications including pelvic inflammatory disease (PID) and sexually transmitted diseases (STDs).

- If prone to vaginitis, take with you one small bag each of boric acid capsules and acidophilus caps (or just the boric acid and buy yogurt locally).

WEST NILE VIRUS

WNV is mosquito-borne and is found in temperate and tropical areas of the world, which, since the mid-1990s, has spread globally. This year, the U.S. experienced one of its worst epidemics. About 80% of those infected will show no symptoms. Up to 20% have mild symptoms: fever, body aches, headache, fatigue, nausea and vomiting, swollen lymph nodes, a skin rash on the stomach, back, and chest, and muscle weakness and numbness. They last from a few days to a few weeks.

HOMEOPATHY

We have not treated any cases of WNV and found little in the homeopathic literature. Based on the symptoms, try one of these two medicines:

- *Arsenicum album* (Arsenic): Watery nasal discharge, Nausea, vomiting, restlessness. Great thirst to drink sips of cold water.

- **Gelsemium** (Yellow jasmine): Dizzy, drowsy, droopy, and dull. Flu-like.

PREVENTION

- Take mosquito-repellant precautions such as staying indoors at dusk, using screens, and avoiding marshes or stagnant pools of water.

- Use mosquito repellants, preferably with less than 10% DEET, or aromatic herbal repellants, such as oil of lemon eucalyptus, or *Citronella*, (this may interfere with homeopathic medicines and should not be used on children under the age of three), but is effective against mosquitoes. (See INSECT BITES AND STINGS , page 161 and Malaria, page 173.)

- Use permethrin on clothing, shoes, bed nets, and camping gear.

- Apply repellants only to exposed areas, not under clothing. Do not apply to eyes or mouth, and apply sparingly around the ears. To apply repellant to your face, spray on hands, then apply to face.

- Do not use any more repellant than necessary.

- Once you are indoors, wash your skin well with soap and water, especially if you have used repeated applications of repellants.

MORE NATURAL TIPS

- Turmeric (*Curcumin*) has been shown to be effective against WNV.

- Neem oil has been shown to be an effective mosquito repellent.

- Soy oil (preferably non-GMO) repellents appear to be as effective as DEET.

- Catnip oil, in Iowa University experiments, was shown to be as much as ten percent more effective than DEET.

- Repel, a repellent containing lemon eucalyptus, has been shown to last longer than DEET and is widely available. (It may decrease the effectiveness of single-dose homeopathic medicines due to its aromatic properties.)

LIFESAVERS

- A small number of people have died of WNV. If you are going to an area where this is an outbreak or epidemic, use a repellant. Encephalitis and meningitis are serious complications.

W

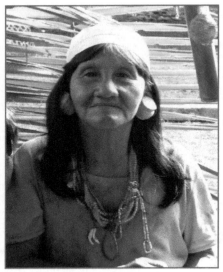

Huaorani chief Moi's mother, Ecuadorian Amazon

ANSWERS TO HOMEOPATHIC PRACTICE CASES

1. Burn: *Cantharis*
2. Food Poisoning: *Ipecac.*
3. Insect Bite: *Apis*
4. Bladder Infection: *Sarsaparilla*
5. Acute Appendicitis: *Bryonia*
6. Traveler's Diarrhea: *Podophyllum*
7. Cold: *Allium cepa*
8. Ear Infection *Chamomilla*
9. Airplane Anxiety: *Aconite*
10. Hay Fever: *Sabadilla*

BIBLIOGRAPHY

HOMEOPATHY BOOKS

Perko, Sandra J. *The Homeopathic Treatment of Influenza-Special Bird Flu* Edition: Surviving Epidemics and Pandemics, Past, Present and Future With Homeopathy. San Antonio: Benchmark Homeopathic Publications, 2005.

Fascinating account of how homeopathy worked effectively in the influenza pandemic.

Reichenberg-Ullman, Judyth. *Whole Woman Homeopathy: A Safe, Natural, Effective Alternative to Drugs, Hormones, and Surgery.* Edmonds: Picnic Point Press, 2005, 2014.

Ullman, Robert and Judyth Reichenberg. *Homeopathic Self-Care: The Quick and Easy Guide to the Whole Family.* Edmonds: Picnic Point Press, 2013.

Our tried-and-true, comprehensive, full-size, homeopathic self-care book with over 70 conditions. Has sold over 20,000 copies. Companion self-care kit.

Ullman, Robert and Judyth Reichenberg. *The Patient's Guide to Homeopathic Medicine.* Edmonds: Picnic Point Press, 2000.

What patients need to know to make the most of their homeopathic care.

TRAVEL HEALTH BOOKS

Hatt, John. *The Tropical Traveller, The Essential Guide to Travel in Hot Countries.* London: Penguin Books Ltd., 1993.

Invaluable information about staying healthy while living in the tropics.

Kramer, Susan. *The Healthy Traveler: A Handbook of Easy Solutions for Common Travel Ailments.* Atlanta: Aspen Press, 2002.

Common-sense advice from an herbalist.

Lessell, Colin. *The World Travellers' Manual of Homeopathy.* Essex: CWD Daniel Company, Ltd., 2004.

Good for homeopaths. Obscure diseases.

Lichten, Joanne. *How to Stay Healthy & Fit on the Road*. Houston: Nutrifit Publishing, 2001. Fun, practical.
Written by a high-power dietician/speaker/traveler.

Lorie, Jonathan, Editor. *The Traveler's Handbook: The Insider's Guide to World Travel*. Guildford: The Globe Pequot Press, 2000.
Comprehensive, practical, and encyclopedic. Useful for ambitious, far-flung travel or residency.

Pitt, Richard. *The Natural Medicine Guide for Travel and Home*. Haren, Netherlands: Homeolinks, 2013.
Excellent, informative, well-researched. Extensive information on homeopathic treatment of tropical diseases, especially in Africa and Asia.

Roy, Ravi and Carola Lage-Roy. *The Homeopathic Guide for Travelers: Remedies for Health and Safety*. Berkeley: North Atlantic, 2010.
Popular in Germany. Much useful information.

Werner, David, Carol Thuman, and James Maxwell. *Where There Is No Doctor: Village Health Care Handbook*. Berkeley: Hesperian Health Guides, 2013.
Invaluable classic. The most widely used health care manual for health workers for the past 25 years. Translated into more than 75 languages.

Wise, Mark. *The Travel Doctor: Your guide to staying healthy while you travel*. London: Firefly Books, 2002.
An excellent, information-packed book from a well-traveled, experienced medical doctor.

Young, Isabelle. *Lonely Planet Healthy Travel Central & South America*. Melbourne: Lonely Planet Publications, 2000.
Compact, user-friendly.

VACCINATION

CDC Health Information for International Travel 2014: *The Yellow Book.* Northampton: Oxford University Press, 2013.

Conventional view of travel vaccines.

Eisenstein, Mayer. *Make an Informed Vaccine Decision for the Health of Your Child: A Parent's Guide to Childhood Shots.* Santa Fe: New Atlantean Press, 2010.

Up-to-date, informative.

Neustaedter, Randall. *The Vaccine Guide: Risks and Benefits for Children and Adults.* Berkeley: North Atlantic Press, 2002.

Detailed information about vaccinations from the point of view of a homeopath.

INDEX

ABOUT THE AUTHORS: THE SAVVY TRAVEL DOCS

Judyth Reichenberg-Ullman, N.D., M.S.W., and Robert Ullman, N.D., are licensed naturopathic physicians board certified in homeopathy. Authors of eight books on homeopathic medicine, including the best-selling *Ritalin-Free Kids*, they have been columnists for the *Townsend Letter for Doctors* since 1990, and have taught homeopaths throughout the U.S. and internationally.

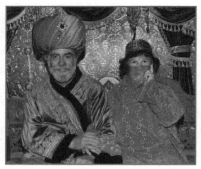

The Ullmans practice at The Northwest Center for Homeopathic Medicine in Edmonds, Washington. As classical homeopaths, they specialize in treating adults with mental and emotional problems, in addition to offering a general homeopathic practice. Dr. Reichenberg-Ullman also specializes in natural women's health care. Dr. Ullman is internationally known for his work with children

Sultan and Sultana. Cistern, Istanbul

with behavioral, learning, and developmental problems. Both doctors offer Travel Well natural health consultations. The doctors treat patients by telephone and video consultation, as well as in person. They have an international practice. Dr. Reichenberg-Ullman is fluent in English, Spanish and French. The doctors can be reached by email at drreichenberg@gmail.com and drbobullman@gmail.com.

The couple loves to travel, and has visited over 40 countries (Judyth is a Top Contributor to Trip Advisor) over as many years. They also enjoy hiking, gardening, kayaking, yoga, meditation, sacred and world music, and the Dances of Universal Peace. They live in Langley, Washington, on Whidbey Island, and in Pucón, Chile, with their golden retrievers and farm animals.

Please visit www.healthyhomeopathy.com or call (425) 774-5599.

 healthy Homeopathy

Order Your Homeopathic Self-Care Medicine Kit Today!

The 50 Most Useful Homeopathic Medicines for First Aid and Acute Illnesses Recommended in Our Book:
Homeopathic Self-Care:
The Quick and Easy Guide for the Whole Family

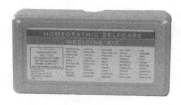

Small, Lightweight, Inexpensive.
Perfect for Home, Camping and Travel!

5 ½" long, 3" wide and 1 ¾ " high, it comes shrink-wrapped and weighs only 1 lb. Remedies are in tiny 30C potency pellets, enough doses in a small vial to last for years. Refills available for frequently used remedies.

Aconite	*Gelsemium*	*Podophyllum*
Allium cepa	*Glonoine*	*Pulsatilla*
Argentum nitricum	*Hepar sulph*	*Rhus tox*
Apis	*Hypericum*	*Rumex*
Arnica	*Ignatia*	*Ruta*
Arsenicum album	*Ipecac*	*Sarsaparilla*
Belladonna	*Kali bichromicum*	*Sepia*
Bryonia	*Lachesis*	*Silica*
Carbo veg	*Ledum*	*Spongia tosta*
Chamomilla	*Lycopodium*	*Staphysagria*
China	*Magnesia phos*	*Sulphur*
Cocculus	*Mercurius*	*Symphytum*
Coffea	*Natrum mur*	*Tabacum*
Colocynthis	*Nux vomica*	*Urtica urens*
Drosera	*Petroleum*	*Veratrum album*
Euphrasia	*Phosphorus*	
Ferrum phos	*Phytolacca*	

Order from www.healthyhomeopathy.com or call Northwest Center for Homeopathic Medicine (425) 774-5599